THE THRILL OF
KRILL

THE THRILL OF
KRILL

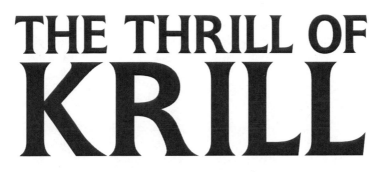

What You Should Know
About Krill Oil

Dennis Goodman, MD, FACC

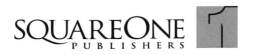

SQUAREONE
PUBLISHERS

The information and advice contained in this book are based upon the research and the personal and professional experiences of the author. They are not intended as a substitute for professional healthcare advice. The publisher and author are not responsible for any adverse effects or consequences resulting from the use of any of the suggestions, preparations, or procedures discussed in this book. All matters pertaining to your physical health should be supervised by a healthcare professional. It is a sign of wisdom, not cowardice, to seek a second or third opinion.

COVER DESIGNER: Jeannie Tudor
TYPESETTER: Gary A. Rosenberg

Square One Publishers
115 Herricks Road
Garden City Park, NY 11040
(516) 535-2010 • (877) 900-BOOK
www.squareonepublishers.com

Library of Congress Cataloging-in-Publication Data

Goodman, Dennis (Dennis A.), author.
  The thrill of krill : what you should know about krill oil / Dennis Goodman, MD, FACC.
      pages cm
  Includes bibliographical references and index.
    ISBN 978-0-7570-0418-6 (pbk.) — ISBN 978-0-7570-0419-3 (hardback)
  1. Krill oil—Health aspects. 2. Krill oil—Therapeutic use. 3. Marine oils in human nutrition. 4. Dietary supplements. I. Title.
    RM666.K75G66   2015
    615.3'4—dc23
                                                        2015001918

Printed in the United States of America

10   9   8   7   6   5   4   3   2   1

Contents

Acknowledgments, ix

Introduction, 1

1. Dealing with Health Conditions, 5

2. Sources of Omega-3s, 23

3. All About Krill, 39

4. Fighting Cardiovascular Disease, 49

5. Relieving Joint Pain, 69

6. Dealing with Women's Health, 85

7. Alleviating Depression, 97

8. Additional Health Benefits, 111

9. Krill Oil Guidelines, 125

Conclusion, 137

References, 139

About the Author, 151

Index, 153

To Wendy Fisher,
for her constant love, passion,
and encouragement.

Acknowledgments

I am deeply appreciative of those who have nurtured, guided, mentored, and supported me throughout my life. Without these wonderful people, this book would not be possible.

I would like to thank my parents, Joe and Muriel Goodman, for inspiring me to always be kind and caring, to be my best self, and for ensuring that I received the very finest education in South Africa—which culminated in the conferment of my medical degree from one of the best universities in the world—the University of Cape Town, South Africa.

Many thanks go to my teachers and mentors in high school and medical school. There is a long list of people to whom I am grateful, but I especially want to acknowledge Norman Sandler; Elliot Wolf; Eddie Tannenbaum; Doc Thomas; and Professors Stuart Saunders, Lionel Opie, Leo Schamroth, Cecil Craig, and Jannie Louw. I was privileged to do my internship at Groote Schuur Hospital in Cape Town, where the first heart transplant was performed by Christian Barnard in 1967. During those years in medical school and during my internship, away from my hometown of Johannesburg, four wonderful families took me in as one of their own; for this, I thank Dr. Louis and Joan Abramowitz, Harry and Myra Mark, Harry and Pauline Stein, and Dov and Bernice Borok, and all their children.

I would like to thank Dr. Philip Troen and Dr. Sheldon Adler of Montefiore Hospital in Pittsburgh, for giving me the opportunity to do my internal medicine residency in the United States and subsequently become a citizen of this great country.

Thanks also to Dr. Robert Roberts, chief of the cardiology department at Baylor College of Medicine, which is associated with Dr. Michael Debakey's cardiac surgery program in Houston, Texas. At Baylor, I received the very best cardiology training. Special thanks to my mentors, Drs. Al Raizner, John Lewis, Jim Young, Craig Pratt, Mario Verani, Phil Henry, Miguel Quinones, William Zoghbi, and the Chapman group.

I would like to thank all my colleagues and friends at Scripps Memorial Hospital and Scripps Clinic—Drs. John Backman, Isaac Bakst, Neil and Ruth Berkowitz, Joel Bernstein, Mark Boiskin, Barry Broomberg, Maurice Buchbinder, Stephen Capon, Martin Charlat, David Dockweiler, Dan Einhorn, Shaun Evans, Ray and Rhona Fink, Carl Fricks, Martin Griglak, Fred Hanson, Wayne Hooper, Paul Hyde, Len Jurkowski, Elizabeth Kaback, Norman Kane, Jurgen Lenz, John Lischke, Mike Mahdavi, Scott McCaul, Lou Katzman, Marc Kramer, Barnie Meltzer, Chris Mende, Frank Meyer, Howard Miller, Ernie Pund, Simon Ritchken, Don Ritt, David Roseman, Mark Sedwitz, Lorna Swartz, Paul Tierstein, Doug Triffon, Sabina Wallach, Pat Wolcott, and the great cardiac surgeons Scott Brewster, Don Buehler, Sasha Giritsky, Richard Stahl, Demetrio Vasquez, and so many others. I particularly want to thank Dr. John Carson, an exceptional human being who exemplifies the values, virtues, and teachings of Sir William Osler.

A special thanks to Gary Fybel, the administrator of Scripps Memorial, and to Susan Taylor, for their enduring friendship and support. Thank you to Irma Flores and Suzi Bustamante for all their help during my tenure as Chief of Cardiology at Scripps Memorial. And many thanks to my incredible office manager, Debbie Heggins, and nurse practitioner, Robin Whitman, who worked with me for over twenty years.

Thanks to Mimi Guarnieri and Rauni King, who put me on the path to becoming a truly integrative physician. I learned so much from them and their great team at Scripps Center for Integrative Medicine. And thanks to Debbie Shainfeld and Deedee Sides for their passionate commitment to integrative health.

My thanks also go to Drs. Glenn Fishman and Norma Keller,

who gave me the opportunity to work and teach as a cardiologist at one of the great medical institutions of the world, New York University Langone Medical Center. Thanks to the great staff and my previous partners at New York Medical Associates, Drs. Mark Lipton, Stanley Schrem, and Jeffrey Kohn. Thank you to Dr Steve Lamm and all the wonderful physicians and staff at the Preston R. Tisch Center for Men's Health, NYU, where I am privileged to work. I am indebted to Drs. Frank Lipman, Daryl Isaacs, Lionel Bissoon, Keith Berkowitz, Leah Lagos, and Marnie Potash for their unwavering support.

Thanks to the staff at Square One Publishers—to my publisher, Rudy Shur, who has been the Rock of Gibraltar with his wisdom and support throughout the process, and to my fabulous editors, Marie Caratozzolo, Joanne Abrams, and Miye Bromberg for their hard work and dedication to this project. My sincere gratitude to Liza Burby for being such an incredible resource.

I thank Drs. Norman Kane, Norman Gordon, Mike Forman, and Jim Adams; Gershon Jaffe; Mike, Patti, and Russel Hoffman; Reuben Klamer; Dennis and Rosa Basson; Marty Katz; Michael Moffson; Linda Mirels and Gerard Mosse; Philip Kirsh and Monette de Botton; Hilton Mirels and Val Schaer; Barry Stiefel; Mark Rosenberg; Barry and Anne Stein; Dean Draznin; Terri Slater; David Shalev; Rabbi and Marsha Tanzer; and Rabbi and Adina Shippel for providing a wealth of knowledge and friendship.

Huge thanks to my special partner, Wendy Fisher, who has encouraged and supported me through the many hours of researching and writing this book. Thanks to my sisters, Myra Salkinder and Elaine Lucey, and to all of my family. I am so fortunate to have their constant love and support.

Enormous thanks to my incredible children—Adam and my daughter-in-law Anat, Jonathan, and Rebecca—as well as to their wonderful mother, Tanya. Additional thanks to Adam and Jonathan for all their editing and research help along the way.

Lastly, I want to thank all of the patients I have treated over my twenty-five years in practice. They have given me so much pleasure and the greatest gift of all—a meaningful life and the opportunity to make a small difference in the world.

Introduction

Imagine a natural supplement that is able to do the following:

- Protect against cardiovascular disease and stroke.
- Lower blood pressure and cholesterol.
- Reduce arthritis pain.
- Moderate premenstrual discomfort.
- Relieve symptoms of menopause.
- Alleviate depression.
- Combat dementia.
- Slow down the aging process.

As a practicing physician specializing in cardiology and integrative medicine, I dedicate a great deal of my time to validating or refuting such statements, which are often made by neutraceutical companies. I feel it is my responsibility to research and find out as much as I can about a particular supplement before recommending it to my patients—or before taking it myself. When it comes to the omega-3 fatty acids, there has been large body of scientific research to sift through. But in doing so, I have been convinced that these beneficial fats have met my high standards for recommendation, and that krill oil is the best and safest way to obtain them. In this book, I have shared my findings with you.

To best safeguard your health, being proactive is key. Along with having annual checkups, it's important to eat a healthy diet and exercise regularly. What is perhaps just as important is listening to your body—after all, you know it better than anyone else. Whenever there is a health concern, seek medical help and educate yourself on the condition. By understanding the problem and by becoming aware of its symptoms and underlying cause (or causes), you will become better equipped to take control and actually do something to help yourself.

While making positive lifestyle changes can drastically improve the quality of your life, science has also shown that the right nutrients can help treat, reverse, and even prevent many serious diseases and health conditions. And that is exactly what I hope to show you in this book. I am a strong supporter of natural alternatives, which tend to be well-tolerated and "do no harm." Pharmaceutical drugs have a legitimate place, but in many cases, natural alternatives may work just as well, and without negative side effects.

Throughout my career, I have researched and studied over one-hundred nutrients. Among the important lessons I've learned is that just because a nutritional supplement (or anything you put in your mouth) is natural and supposedly "does no harm," it is not necessarily good for you. Before I am convinced of the merits of a nutrient, I always have three questions in mind:

■ Is there enough clinical evidence (that is, well-conducted research studies) that shows a beneficial effect? Is it sufficient enough to recommend the nutrient to my patients and to take it myself?
■ Is the evidence consistent and robust enough to conclude that the nutrient has proven benefits?
■ Is it safe? Does it have any significant side effects?

For decades, medical researchers have extolled the many health benefits of the essential fatty acids known as omega-3s.

Vital to the optimal functioning of virtually every cell, organ, and system in our bodies, omega-3s help keep our systems in balance. Because the body cannot manufacture them in adequate amounts, we must obtain these "good fats" through diet and supplements. While fish oil has long been viewed as the best omega-3 supplement, I have discovered that there is now an even better alternative—oil sourced from tiny ocean-dwelling crustaceans called krill. I have written *The Thrill of Krill* to share this important discovery with you.

Designed to provide a clear understanding of the benefits and uses of supplemental krill oil, *The Thrill of Krill* opens with informative chapters on the role of omega-3s in improving and sustaining good health. Included is a breakdown of these essential nutrients along with a brief look at their use throughout history, which dates as far back as the ancient Romans, who reserved this "health elixir" for soldiers and nobility. As the various natural sources of these healthful fats are presented, you will learn how the oil from ocean-dwelling krill is a superior source—and discover how something that is such a tiny part of the vast ocean can have such a dramatic impact on good health.

Chapters that follow focus on the proven effectiveness of krill oil and its rich omega-3 content on treating (and even preventing in some cases) a number of common, often debilitating health problems. Included are its role in fighting such serious cardiovascular conditions such as atherosclerosis, coronary heart disease, high blood pressure, and stroke, as well as its effectiveness in reducing the painful symptoms of rheumatoid and osteoarthritis. The chapter on women's health covers the management of such significant conditions as premenstrual syndrome, dysmenorrhea (painful menstruation), and menopause. It also presents the importance of omega-3s during pregnancy and lactation—for both mother and child. Krill oil's role in managing depression and treating neurological-based disorders like attention deficit hyperactivity disorder (ADHD), dementia, and Alzheimer's disease is discussed, as is its effectiveness in reducing chronic inflammation and the broad spectrum of disorders it can cause or exacerbate, such as lupus, asthma, inflammatory bowel disease, and cancer.

High levels of the omega-3s found in krill oil have also been associated with a slower progression of the aging process itself—and its wide spectrum of age-related disorders.

A solid foundation of medical research has long supported the extensive health benefits of omega-3 fatty acids. With krill oil as a superior source of these valuable nutrients, I hope you consider making them—along with a healthy diet and lifestyle—part of your daily regimen for overall fitness and well-being.

1

Dealing with
Health Conditions

When facing any type of health concern, from a simple headache or aching joints to more serious issues like high blood pressure or a heart condition, most people head for the medicine cabinet. It's how we've been conditioned. There are, of course, times when there is no other choice than to treat certain problems with pharmaceuticals, whether they are over-the-counter treatments or a doctor's prescribed drugs. It is well-documented, however, that when it comes to using medications, our bodies don't get something for nothing. We've all heard those commercials touting the benefits of a drug that promises life-changing results, only to be followed by its potential side effects—typically mentioned with the rapid-fire speech of an auctioneer. The fact is, every drug comes with a downside (often, more than one), which can be as mild as occasional dizziness or nausea, or as serious as coma or even death. No wonder more and more people are choosing to treat their ailments with natural alternatives like vitamins, herbs, and other dietary supplements.

What is just as distressing as the additional health issues caused by a medication's side effects is the fact that although the drug may reduce or eliminate the symptoms it is meant to treat, it doesn't necessarily resolve the underlying condition. There is, of course, a legitimate place for certain drugs, which should *always* be taken under the guidance of a healthcare professional. As a physician, I am always weighing the benefits versus the risks of any prescribed medication or procedure. Increasingly, however, doctors are becoming more accepting of natural alternatives. For the most part, these supplements tend to be well-tolerated and do "no harm," and many have been proven effective in treating a variety of conditions. I have dedicated myself to studying these natural alternatives, and have been impressed by many of my findings. Among the most effective and powerful of these core nutrients, which have been scientifically proven to provide abundant medical benefits, are the omega-3 fatty acids.

Essential to the optimal functioning of virtually every cell, organ, and system in our bodies, omega-3s help keep our systems in balance. Because the body cannot manufacture adequate amounts of these fats, we must obtain them through diet and natural supplements.

Research has shown that maintaining the body's natural balance of the right omega-3s may improve or even prevent a broad spectrum of debilitating disorders and conditions, in particular those caused by inflammation; cardiovascular disease; poor memory; cognitive decline; and autoimmune disorders. They also have positive effects on hormone-related issues like thyroid conditions, depression, and mood swings. Later chapters will detail the potential healing power of omega-3s on these and other health problems.

In summary, omega-3s offer multiple benefits for good health, and have been associated with the following:

- Reducing the risk of heart attack and stroke.

- Lowering elevated triglyceride levels.

- Alleviating depression.

- Reducing the inflammation associated with asthma.

- Curbing the stiffness and joint pain of arthritis.

- Protecting against Alzheimer's disease and dementia.

- Slowing the gradual memory loss due to aging.

- Playing an important role in the visual and neurological development in infants.

- Reducing the symptoms of ADHD in some children.

- Benefitting skin health—reducing wrinkles and controlling conditions like psoriasis.

- Increasing the effectiveness of anti-inflammatory medications, as well as antidepressants.

As you will see, while a lack of omega-3s can bring about a number of health issues, restoring proper levels can help the body resolve them. Even more important, maintaining appropriate levels can play a part in the prevention of these conditions and the maintenance of good health.

Before going further, it's important to first understand more about dietary fat with a focus on omega-3s.

DIETARY FAT—THE GOOD AND THE BAD

When most people think of a high-fat diet, they associate it with serious health risks, from obesity and diabetes to inflammation and heart disease. Interestingly, Americans consume less total fat today than they did in the 1960s, yet rates of obesity and heart disease are higher—and continue to climb. According to recent studies, one reason is the dietary increase of high-glycemic carbohydrates, which cause insulin resistance and heighten the risk of obesity, diabetes, and heart disease. High intake of refined sugars, which are contained in soft drinks, candy, baked goods, and other sweets, is also strongly associated with high triglycerides (fats in the blood).

When it comes to fats, the focus has shifted to the *type* that is eaten, not the quantity. The right fats, when consumed in moderation, are an essential component of a well-rounded, healthy diet. Knowing the "good" fats from the "bad" will help you make smarter dietary choices and, as a result, maintain good health.

Saturated Fats

The main dietary cause of high cholesterol and unhealthy weight gain, saturated fats are found primarily in fatty animal proteins such as beef and pork, as well as full-fat dairy products like whole milk, butter, and cheese. They are typically solid at room temperature. Due to the detrimental effect of saturated fats on overall health, reducing their consumption is strongly recommended. Choose lean meats and reduced-fat dairy products, and cook with healthier oils, such as olive oil and vegetable-based oils.

Trans Fats

Also known as *trans-fatty acids*, trans fats are produced when vegetable oils are hydrogenated to make them more solid and stable. The hydrogenation process also prolongs the oil's shelf life, which is why trans fats are often used to make processed foods, fast foods, commercial baked goods, and solid margarine. In the recent past, many food manufacturers have taken steps to remove this ingredient from their products, as scientists have discovered that trans fats from partially hydrogenated oils are even more harmful than saturated fats. They increase the level of low-density lipoproteins (LDLs)—the "bad" cholesterol—while decreasing high-density lipoproteins (HDLs)—the "good" cholesterol. (For more information, see the inset "Cholesterol" on page 12.)

We must try to avoid trans fats at all costs by staying away from commercially prepared baked items (cakes, cookies, donuts, muffins, etc.), solid margarine, and foods that are fried in partially hydrogenated oils. When buying packaged foods, be sure to check nutrition labels. If the product contains partially hydrogenated oil, it also contains trans fats and should be avoided.

Unsaturated Fats

Coming primarily from vegetable and marine sources, unsaturated fats tend to be liquid at room temperature. They consist of monounsaturated fats and polyunsaturated fats, which are both considered "good" fats. Keep in mind, however, that all fats—both good and bad—are dense in calories, so even unsaturated fats should be consumed in moderation.

Monounsaturated Fats

Healthy monounsaturated fats reduce LDL levels without causing a negative impact on HDL cholesterol. They also provide nutrients to help keep the body's cells healthy. Foods high in monounsaturated fats include a number of plant-based oils, such as olive, canola, peanut, safflower, and sesame oils. Avocados, peanuts, macadamia nuts, and hazelnuts are other rich sources.

Polyunsaturated Fats

Essential for good health, polyunsaturated fats lower LDL cholesterol and triglycerides. Like monounsaturated fats, they also provide nutrients to help maintain the body's cells. Two groups in particular, omega-3 and omega-6, must be obtained through the diet, as they are not adequately produced by the body. Omega-6 fats are plentiful in a number of foods, from nuts and seeds to vegetable oils, so most people consume sufficient amounts without even trying. Omega-3s, on the other hand, are not as abundant. They are found mainly in fatty fish like salmon, herring, and trout, which contain the beneficial "long-chain" fatty acids EPA and DHA. The suggested dietary intake of this type of fish is three times a week. (It must also be noted that cooking fish at high temperatures breaks down a high proportion of EPA and DHA.)

Krill—tiny shrimp-like crustaceans—are another very rich source of EPA and DHA, as well as phospholipids and highly potent antioxidants. The oil sourced from krill is available as a superior supplement. Other sources of omega-3s are discussed in detail in the next chapters. For additional information on the Omega Groups, see page 10.

Understanding the variation among fats is an important step towards achieving a wholesome diet. Including the right amount of good fat while reducing consumption of saturated fats and eliminating trans fats are keys to good health. Also keep in mind that in addition to bad fats, unhealthy levels of triglycerides and cholesterol are influenced by an excessive intake of sugar and processed foods. Avoiding or drastically reducing your intake of these foods is strongly recommended.

When choosing oils for dressing salads and preparing low-heat dishes, olive, flaxseed, and canola oils should be your primary selections. For high-heat cooking, choose oils like sunflower, safflower, canola, peanut, and macadamia, which have high smoke points. This means they are able to withstand higher temperatures without breaking down, allowing food to cook more quickly and absorb less oil.

THE OMEGA GROUPS

Although a low-fat diet is generally considered healthier than one that is high in fat, our bodies require a certain amount of fat for proper growth and functioning. Like vitamins and minerals, a number of these fats either cannot be manufactured by the body or are unable to be produced in adequate amounts. Often referred to as "essential," these beneficial nutrients, which are found among the omega-3 and omega-6 fatty acid groups, must be obtained through diet or supplements.

Omega-3 fatty acids (also known as *n*-3 fatty acids) are polyunsaturated. They have been shown to reduce inflammation and help prevent chronic diseases, such as heart disease and arthritis. They are also important for brain health, as well as normal growth and development. The three major types are eicosapentaenoic acid, docosahexaenoic acid, and alpha-linolenic acid.

Eicosapentaenoic acid (EPA) has been found to have a positive effect on coronary heart disease, and in reducing high triglyceride levels, high blood pressure, and inflammation. It is found in krill and fatty cold-water fish like salmon, cod, herring, mackerel, and sardines. *Docosahexaenoic acid* (DHA) is good for your heart, as well as a healthy brain. Like EPA, it is found in krill and fatty cold-water fish. *Alpha-linolenic acid* (ALA) has been shown to reduce inflammation and prevent chronic diseases. Dietary sources are plant based and include dark green leafy vegetables like kale and spinach, Brussels sprouts, soybeans, and walnuts. Oils such as soy, canola, and flaxseed are other sources. The body is able to convert only a small amount of ALA into EPA and DHA. Therefore, even if foods containing ALA are consumed in large quantities, it would still not be enough to get your recommended intake.

Like the omega-3s, omega-6 fatty acids (also known as *n*-6 fatty acids) are polyunsaturated fats. Along with omega-3s, they are important for proper brain functioning (especially during early development) and the body's normal growth and development. They also play a role in stimulating skin and hair growth, maintaining healthy bones, and regulating metabolism. The main types of omega-6 fats are linoleic acid, gamma-linolenic acid, and arachidonic acid.

Linoleic acid comes primarily from plant-based oils, including safflower, corn, sunflower, and soybean. They are also plentiful in seeds and nuts, particularly sunflower seeds, pine nuts, and pecans. A small amount is found in milk and certain cheeses, like brie, blue, and Swiss. *Gamma-linolenic acid* (GLA) is found in borage oil, black currant oil, and evening primrose oil. *Arachidonic acid* (AA) comes primarily from meats and other animal products, including egg yolks.

Although omega-6 fats are beneficial in small amounts, too much (particularly arachidonic acid) can lead to chronic inflammation and a number of other health problems. For general good health, the intake of omega-6 fats and omega-3s should be in a proper ratio—between 3:1 and 6:1. Unfortunately, Americans tend to consume significantly more omega-6 fats than they need—for the standard American diet, that ratio is between 10:1 and 25:1. It's important to decrease the intake of omega-6s, while increasing the intake of omega-3s.

Another omega group—the omega-9 fatty acids—are monounsaturated fats that offer a variety of health benefits. Shown to increase beneficial HDL cholesterol and decrease harmful LDL cholesterol, omega-9s are important for heart health. *Oleic acid* is the main type of omega-9 commonly found in oils like canola and safflower. Unlike omega-3 and omega-6 fatty acids, the body is able to produce omega-9s in adequate amounts, which are also beneficial when obtained from food sources.

All of the omega fatty acids, in proper amounts, are important for overall good health and nutrition.

OMEGA-3s AT THE CELLULAR LEVEL

One of the reasons omega-3 fatty acids are considered beneficial is their role in cells. Every human cell has a protective, two-layer permeable membrane called the *lipid bilayer* or *phospholipid bilayer.*

Cholesterol

Cholesterol is a soft, waxy substance that is found in the bloodstream and carried through the body in lipoprotein particles. It is both made by the body and consumed in animal foods. Although your body needs cholesterol, the intake of too much can clog your arteries, which means your heart will receive less blood and oxygen. This can result in serious cardiovascular problems.

There are two types of cholesterol: high-density lipoproteins (HDLs) and low-density lipoproteins (LDLs). LDLs are known as "bad" (or "lousy") cholesterol because they can form as plaque along your arteries and increase your risk of heart disease. HDLs, on the other hand, are considered "good" (or "happy") cholesterol, whose main job is to collect, break down, and excrete the LDLs that are already in the body.

Therefore, your goal for optimal health should include a low LDL count and a high HDL count. Ideally, your total cholesterol (LDL plus HDL) should be under 200 milligrams per deciliter (mg/dL) and your HDL should be over 40 milligrams per deciliter (mg/dL).

If your cholesterol is high or has a sudden increase, adjusting your dietary habits is critical. Although a portion of cholesterol is due to heredity, limiting your intake of "bad" cholesterol foods is an important step in keeping the levels under control and lowering your risk for serious illness.

Each layer is made primarily of proteins, cholesterol, and fats in the form of phospholipids. Phospholipids are similar to triglycerides except that one of the three fatty acid units has been replaced with a molecule that contains phosphorus. These fats make up the structural component of the cell membranes, keeping them flexible and permeable. Maintaining this permeability is important so that nutrients are able to pass through the membranes into the cells. It also allows waste products to pass out of the cells. This is one of the reasons omega-3s, which have a flexible, long-chain structure, are so beneficial. They keep the cell membranes fluid and stable, preventing them from becoming too stiff and rigid for nutrients and waste to pass in and out as needed.

The type of fat you consume determines the type of fatty acid found in the cell membranes. A diet that is high in cholesterol and consisting mostly of saturated fat and trans-fatty acids results in cell membranes that tend to be rigid and less permeable than those found in a person whose diet includes optimal levels of unsaturated fatty acids.

Research has shown that the central factor in the development of virtually every disease is an alteration in cell membrane function. Without the right type of fats, cell membranes lose their ability to hold water and vital nutrients. And without healthy membranes, cells simply cannot function properly. They lose their ability to communicate with other cells and to be controlled by regulating hormones.

High levels of unhealthy fatty acids are also toxic. When this occurs, cells typically isolate them as phospholipids within the membranes. When stimulated, however, the fatty acids may be released, provoking a harmful inflammatory response from the body's immune system.

Omega-3 fats form an integral part of cell membranes that affects the optimal function of cell receptors. In addition to maintaining the structure of healthy cell membranes, omega-3s serve as the starting point for making hormones that regulate multiple body functions including blood clotting and inflammation. They also bind to cell receptors that regulate genetic function.

Scientific researchers have determined that omega-3 fats play an important role in treating as well as reducing the risks of a wide range of diseases and illnesses caused by inflammation. Heart disease, cancer, Alzheimer's disease, and autoimmune disorders including thyroid issues, chronic pain, skin conditions, and lupus are just a few of these health concerns. The positive effects of omega 3s on these and other health concerns will be discussed in detail in later chapters. First, however, it is important to have an understanding of inflammation, which is at the root of most disorders.

INFLAMMATION AND HEALTH

Simply defined, inflammation is the body's natural protective response to an injury, irritation, or harmful pathogen. It is part of our body's defense system—its immune response. When anything harmful or irritating affects a part of the body, the body's biological response is to remove or destroy it. The inflammation that results is actually a sign that the body has begun the healing

Triglycerides

Triglycerides are a type of fat found in the blood and a major source of energy for the body. Excess calories from the food you eat are chemically converted into triglycerides, which are stored in fat cells if they are not used for energy. Hormones can also signal the release of triglycerides from fat cells to provide energy. In normal amounts, triglycerides are vital for good health. However, if you consume more calories than you expend—especially from a diet high in refined sugars and carbohydrates, or one that includes unhealthy fats, like saturated fats and trans fats—your triglyceride level will become too high.

High triglycerides are a major risk factor for heart disease, diabetes and insulin resistance, metabolic syndrome, liver disease, and pancreatitis. Elevated levels also contribute to atherosclerosis (hardening of the arteries), which increases the likelihood of a heart attack or stroke.

process. Be aware that inflammation does not mean infection. Infection is caused by a virus, bacterium, or fungus; inflammation is the body's response to it.

Inflammation can cause an acute or chronic reaction. Acute or short-term inflammation occurs as an immediate response and is quickly resolved. Chronic inflammation is long-term and the cause of numerous illnesses and conditions.

Acute Inflammation

Acute inflammation is the body's immediate response—it's defense reaction—to injuries or to harmful foreign invaders. The affected body part can display any or all of the following symptoms: swelling, redness, heat, pain, and /or loss of function.

Blood flow increases to the affected area, causing warmth and swelling. Pain results from the sensory nerves that are stretched during swelling. Loss of function results from damaged tissue, pain, or joint swelling. Damaged tissue is repaired by white blood cells, which engulf bacteria and other foreign particles.

Acute, short-term inflammation is beneficial. Let's say, for instance, you stub your toe. The tissues swell and the area becomes painful. Your response would be to go easy on that toe and protect it from further injury until the swelling goes down and the pain subsides. The discomfort you feel is like a red flag that keeps you mindful of the injury. This, of course, aids the healing process.

Signs and symptoms of acute inflammation occur quickly and tend to last only a few days, although in some cases they can persist for a few weeks. Some examples of health conditions or situations that can lead to acute inflammation include:

- Sore throat (from a cold or flu)
- Scratch/cut on the skin
- Appendicitis
- Bronchitis
- Dermatitis
- Meningitis (bacterial)
- Sinusitis
- Tonsillitis
- Trauma to the body

Acute inflammation is a natural response that begins the healing process. Under normal circumstances, when anything harmful causes an acute inflammatory response, that inflammation disappears relatively quickly as the affected area heals. If, however, the healing does not occur and the inflammation is continual, the condition becomes chronic, which can lead to much more serious health problems.

Chronic Inflammation

Diseases or health conditions that continue for a long time or recur over and over are considered chronic. Chronic, long-term inflammation is a continual response of the immune system to an ongoing problem—healing does not occur, but low-grade inflammation continues. As explained earlier, stubbing your toe will elicit an acute inflammatory response that will subside as the injury heals, but stubbing that same toe over and over and over again would cause the area more serious harm. In the same way, chronic inflammation, which can last for several months, years, or even a lifetime, can be extremely harmful. A common link to nearly every illness, from diabetes to cancer, chronic inflammation results from a failure to eliminate the cause of acute inflammation.

Keeping in mind that short-term inflammation is part of the healing process, in chronic illnesses, the body continually tries to heal the affected area, which, in turn, can lead to a deterioration of the tissue or a worsening of the condition. Unlike acute inflammation, which is caused by harmful bacteria or a tissue injury, chronic inflammation is caused by certain pathogens, infection with some types of viruses, persistent foreign bodies, or overactive immune system reactions. The outcome is the destruction of tissue, thickening and scarring of connective tissue (fibrosis), or the death of cells or tissues (necrosis).

Chronic inflammation is often painful, as in the case of autoimmune disorders like rheumatoid arthritis, because the swelling pushes against the sensitive nerve endings, which send pain signals to the brain. This can result in stiffness, discomfort, or even debilitation.

Chronic inflammation is not normal nor is it beneficial to the body. It has been implicated as the underlying cause of a number of serious health issues, with autoimmune conditions and heart disease the primary areas of concern.

Autoimmune Disorders

When the body's immune system detects harmful pathogens such as bacteria or viruses, it jumps into action to attack and destroy the unwelcomed intruders. In some cases, the immune system mistakenly views healthy tissues as harmful pathogens and attacks them. Through this misguided reaction, called an *auto-immune response*, the body actually attacks itself. Take type-1 diabetes, for example. Although there is no apparent intruder to fight off, the immune system mistakenly initiates an attack on the insulin-producing cells found in the pancreas. This stops the production of insulin by the body, causing increases in blood glucose. This type of autoimmune disease is commonly found in children and is treated by daily injections.

This harmful response triggers chronic inflammation and is the cause of hundreds of autoimmune diseases. The following list of selected autoimmune disorders indicates in each case how inflammation is involved.

- **Addison's disease.** Inflammation of the adrenal glands.

- **Allergies.** All allergies involve inflammation. For example, with asthma, the airways are inflamed. Hay fever causes inflammation of the membranes of the nose, ear, and throat.

- **Celiac disease.** Inflammation/destruction of the inner lining of the small intestine.

- **Crohn's disease.** Inflammation of the gastrointestinal tract.

- **Lupus.** Inflammation of the joints, lungs, heart, kidney, and skin.

- **Psoriasis.** Inflammation of the skin.

- **Psoriatic arthritis.** Inflammation of joints and the surrounding tissues.

- **Rheumatoid arthritis.** Inflammation of the joints, tissues surrounding the joints, and possibly other organs.

- **Vasculitis.** Inflammation of the blood vessels.

This abbreviated list of autoimmune disorders should serve as an indication of just how common inflammation is in wreaking havoc on good health.

Heart Disease

Chronic inflammation also plays a key role in heart disease, notably in the development and progression of a variety of cardiovascular conditions like coronary atherosclerosis and congestive heart failure. Inflammation is involved in the initiation of plaque buildup, which in turn causes the narrowing of arteries. In Chapter 4, you will find a detailed explanation of this process, which begins when the immune system detects an injury or damage to an arterial wall and then springs into action to heal it.

Unfortunately, chronic inflammation is not always detectable. We may notice the symptoms—and treat them—without getting to the underlying cause. This allows the inflammation to continue and undermine our health.

What does any of this have to do with omega-3s? Later chapters will offer detailed information on their role in improving or preventing specific health issues caused by chronic inflammation, but first, let's take a general look at how they are beneficial.

Omega-3s and Inflammation

A number of scientific studies have strongly indicated that omega-3 fatty acids play an important role in short-circuiting inflammation before it begins—or, at the very least, help resolve the inflammation before it becomes harmful.

One recent study published in the *Proceedings of the National Academy of Sciences* discovered that omega-3 fatty acids inhibit cyclooxygenase 2 (COX-2), an enzyme involved in the production of prostaglandin hormones, which spark inflammation. This reaction is similar to what happens when you take an aspirin or ibuprofen, which disrupts the COX-2 signaling pathway, and causes a reduction of inflammation and pain.

As reported in the *Nature of Chemical Biology*, scientists at the University of Pittsburgh Schools of the Health Sciences published strong evidence that eating foods rich in omega-3 fatty acids or taking omega-3s as a dietary supplement reduces inflammation and lowers the risk of illness and death from cardiovascular and other inflammatory diseases.

The anti-inflammatory activity of omega-3 fatty acids has far-reaching positive effects. It can reduce joint pain, swelling, and stiffness in those who suffer from rheumatoid arthritis and other autoimmune disorders. It plays a part in decreasing high triglyceride levels, and increasing the good HDL cholesterol (which, in turn, helps lower bad LDL cholesterol). It also tends to lower blood pressure in people with hypertension, and helps prevent and treat atherosclerosis by slowing the development of plaque and blood clots, which can clog arteries.

The role of omega-3s in fighting destructive inflammation is nothing short of a miracle, but these fatty acids also play an important role in another area—our hormones.

HORMONAL IMBALANCE

Hormones are the body's chemical messengers. They travel through the bloodstream to control and regulate the activities of certain cells and organs. All of the hormones in your body are designed to interact with each other, and, when in proper balance, they play a part in helping you feel great and experience good health. Essential for growth and development, hormones also have an effect on other bodily functions, including metabolism, mood, sexual function, and reproduction.

A special group of cells known as the endocrine glands produce hormones. These glands, which are located in different areas of the body, secrete hormones into the circulatory system. The hormones then travel through the blood to specific organs or tissues and regulate their activity. The major glands of the endocrine system include the pituitary, hypothalamus, thymus, pineal, testes, ovaries, thyroid, adrenals, parathyroid, and pancreas. Both men and women produce hormones in the same areas with one exception, the sexual organs. Additional male hormones are produced in the testes, while women's are produced in the ovaries.

Like musical notes in a symphony, hormones must work together and interact with each other in perfect harmony. They must also be produced in the appropriate amounts. If your body has too much or too little of a certain hormone, the feedback system will signal the appropriate gland or glands to correct the problem. But if this system has trouble maintaining the right levels, or if your body cannot clear them properly from the bloodstream, hormone imbalance will result—and this can lead to an endocrine disorder or disease.

Endocrine Disorders

There are thousands of different types of endocrine disorders, with diabetes and thyroid conditions among the most common. Of the many thyroid conditions, hypothyroidism and hyperthyroidism are common types. Levels of certain hormones, including those produced by the thyroid, can also be factors in depression and other mood disorders. Let's take a brief look at some of these conditions.

An overactive thyroid that produces too much thyroid hormone is the cause of *hyperthyroidism,* which leads to weight loss, accelerated heart rate, nervousness, and anxiety. Another thyroid issue involving hormone imbalance is *hypothyroidism.* The opposite of hyperthyroidism, this condition is caused by lower production of the thyroid hormone. Its common symptoms include weight gain, fatigue, dry skin, and forgetfulness. Some of these symptoms are also indications of depression.

While thyroid conditions such as hypothyroidism can be factors in depression, research has shown that some symptoms of depression are associated with other hormonal problems, such as those associated with the menstrual cycle. Hormones have also been implicated in *bipolar disorder* or *manic depression*—a mood disorder characterized by episodes of both extreme elation and deep depression.

Although these and other conditions of the endocrine system will be detailed later in the book, it's time for a brief overview on the role of omega-3 fats in their prevention and treatment.

Omega-3s and Hormone Imbalance

As you saw earlier in this chapter, omega-3s are critical for maintaining the structure of healthy cell membranes, keeping them flexible and permeable. In addition to their role at the cellular level, omega-3s also provide the starting point for making hormones. Two of the omega-3 fatty acids—EPA and DHA—are the building blocks for producing hormones that control immune function, and that regulate blood clotting, inflammation, and the contraction and relaxation of artery walls. Without these beneficial fats, the body won't be able to maintain healthy cells, nor will it have what it needs for proper hormone production.

Increasingly, researchers are discovering that omega-3 fatty acids may be effective in alleviating depression and other mood disorders without the dangerous side effects that are typically found with pharmaceutical treatments. Omega-3s have also been effective in preventing cognitive decline, increasing one's attention span, and reducing aggression.

CONCLUSION

A tremendous amount of research has been done on the significant benefits of omega-3 fatty acids, with increasing evidence of their link in the treatment and prevention of a host of illnesses. While this chapter has provided an overview of omega-3s along with a general look at their role in good health, the chapters that follow will offer more specific information.

Along with discovering how vital omega-3s are for good health, you will also learn the best way to obtain them. While fish oil has long been considered the best dietary supplement for these beneficial nutrients, krill oil has proven to be an even better source, a superior choice.

2

Sources of Omega-3s

When most people think of nutrients, they think of vitamins. Although they are vitally important, vitamins are not enough to provide your body with all that it requires to create and maintain optimal health. So what constitutes the complete array of nutrients? To keep our bodies fully functioning, in addition to vitamins, we need minerals, proteins, carbohydrates, water, and lipids (fats and oils). And while we need all of these to sustain health, the problem is that most of us are either unable or unwilling to maintain these nutrients in appropriate amounts. Even worse, by feeding ourselves diets of fast foods, highly processed products, and refined sugars, we are doing more harm to our bodies than good.

An overconsumption of unhealthy fats is a major cause of declining health. Just as problematic is the under-consumption of healthy fats, like the omega-3s. Man has long recognized the benefits of fish oil—a rich source of these beneficial fats. But it is only more recently that scientists have discovered why omega-3s are essential to good health. This chapter begins with a brief history of omega-3s, followed by a discussion of their sources, including one source—krill oil—which has proven to be better than the rest.

HISTORY OF OMEGA-3s

Historians tell us that over 2,000 years ago, the first people to recognize the health benefits of fish oil were the Romans, who reserved this "health elixir" for soldiers and nobility. They placed fish guts in a barrel along with sea water and allowed it to ferment. The unrefined oil that floated to the top was then collected and used. During the Viking Era in the late 700s, fish was a major part of the Norse diet, as was fish liver oil, which came from cod. So valued for its powers of healing and for providing strength and energy, cod liver oil—rich in omega-3 fatty acids—was referred to by the Vikings as "gold of the sea." Along with consuming the oil, Norwegian fishermen commonly rubbed it on their joints and muscles to relieve aches and pains.

By the 1700s, infirmaries were recommending it to relieve a number of illnesses, including rheumatism—a medical condition affecting the joints and connective tissue. Cod liver oil was used as a home remedy for generations since, but it wasn't until the 1950s that medical researchers established its effectiveness in treating ailments like eczema and arthritis. (Anyone who was a child in the 1950s certainly remembers that a spoonful of cod liver oil was promoted by moms everywhere—whether you liked it or not.)

The first pharmaceutical fish oil was produced in 1852 by Peter Möller, a Norwegian pharmacist and entrepreneur. He designed a method for producing a purified form of cod liver oil through a process that involved heating the liver with steam. It took less than an hour for the oil to be skimmed and collected. Called medical cod liver oil, it was sold as a pharmaceutical product. It would be, however, almost another quarter of a century before scientists determined the specific health benefits of fish oils.

The Discovery of Nutritional Fatty Acids

In the early 1900s, dietary fat was viewed simply as a source of calories, interchangeable with carbohydrates. But in 1929, a husband-and-wife team published the first of two papers in the *Journal of Biological Chemistry* that changed this perception. Through their research, George and Mildred Burr discovered the critical connection between fatty acids and health. They were also the ones to coin the phrase "essential fatty acids."

In their 1929 paper, the Burrs presented details of their study, in which they fed young growing rats a fat-free diet. The rats were fed the same amount of food they had been given before the study began, only without the addition of fat. After a number of months, the rats developed scaly skin, sores, and dandruff. Their tails became inflamed, swollen, rigid, and scaly. Their hind paws reddened and sometimes swelled. They also began losing hair, especially around their face and neck. As the rats continued this diet, they began to lose weight and died shortly after. When autopsied, their kidneys and urinary tracts bore significant signs of damage. The Burrs did not know if the rats died because of the missing fats from the diet or from the strain of having to produce the fats internally.

Through their continued research, they made an important discovery. When the rats began showing signs of deterioration, some were given vitamins, which had no effect in reversing the syndrome. Others were given olive oil, lard, linseed oil, or another type of linoleic acid, and began to recover. Continued studies led to the eventual identification of two groups of polyunsaturated fatty acids—omega-6s and omega-3s—as fats that are critical to good health.

Initially, the Burrs' findings were met with controversy. In fact, George Burr received a letter of condolence for coming to the conclusion that fatty acids were beneficial. Even so, future studies, one conducted by George Burr's research assistant, Ralph Holman, demonstrated that linoleic acid was indeed a critical factor in the human diet for good health.

The work the Burrs did opened the floodgates to research in the field of nutritional fatty acids. Since their discovery, researchers have conducted thousands of scientific studies that have validated the connection between the proper balance of fats and good health.

Continued Research

In 1972, groundbreaking research conducted by scientists Hans Olaf Bang and Jørn Dyerberg identified the first connection between omega-3s and cardiovascular health. Their studies were prompted by the observation that the Inuit (Eskimos) of Greenland experienced a very low rate of heart disease. What they found was a connection between the study group's heart health and their diet, which included large quantities of fish, seal, and whale blubber—all rich in the long-chain omega-3s EPA and DHA.

The Seven Country study, initiated by American scientist Ancel Keyes in 1958, examined the relationship between lifestyle and diet (particularly fat composition) to cardiovascular disease and stroke in different countries throughout the world. One of this study's findings suggests that the longevity of the Japanese is due to their higher consumption of fish, rapeseed (source of canola oil), and soya. Among its other findings is that the traditional dietary patterns of Greece, Spain, and Southern Italy—characterized by a proportionally high consumption of olive oil, legumes, unrefined cereals, fruits, and vegetables; moderate-to-high consumption of omega 3-rich fish; moderate consumption of dairy products (mostly as cheese and yogurt); moderate wine consumption; and low consumption of red meat and meat products—have a direct relationship to a lowered risk of cardiovascular problems. Several landmark studies have proven the effectiveness of this healthy style of eating, which has become known as the Mediterranean diet.

Along with the dietary causes of poor cardiovascular health, the study also implicated a number of lifestyle choices, including lack of exercise, smoking, and excessive alcohol consumption. One of the study's promising outcomes indicated that a person can reduce these health risks by making positive dietary and lifestyle changes—regardless of family history.

Although omega-3 fatty acids have been considered essential for normal growth and basic health since the 1930s, an awareness of their additional health benefits has continuously increased dramatically. Recent studies have even included the central role of polyunsaturated fats in brain function. Findings have shown that increased levels of omega-3 acids in tissues correlate with a lowered incidence of some mental illnesses such as depression and of neuro-degenerative diseases like Alzheimer's.

The history of omega-3s and the discovery of its benefits are ongoing, but when a nutrient has managed to help improve human health for more than 2,000 years, it certainly has stood the test of time. The next question is: what is the best way to obtain this precious substance?

OMEGA-3 SOURCES

The main omega-3 fatty acids are found in natural sources—certain plants, animals and animal products, as well as specific types of fish, fish oils, and other forms of marine life. Let's take a closer look at these sources, including areas of concern, such as their purity and bioavailability (the degree to which they are absorbed by the body). For more information on bioavailability, see the inset on page 28.

As seen in Chapter 1, the three major omega-3s are alpha-linolenic acid (ALA), eicosapentaenoic acid (EPA), and docosa-hexaenoic acid (DHA). Of the three, the two long-chain acids—EPA and DHA—are the ones most easily utilized by the body, making them, therefore, the most bioavailable. It is important to know that once consumed, ALA, which comes from plant-based sources, is converted to the more usable EPA and DHA. While this is beneficial, the catch is that only a small percentage is converted, and some is converted to omega-6, a fatty acid that actually triggers inflammation. This means that for optimal omega-3 levels, you also need EPA and DHA, which are found mostly in fatty cold-water fish like salmon, cod, and mackerel, and other forms of marine life, including microalgae (phytoplankton) and tiny crustaceans called krill.

It's time to take a look at the sources of omega-3s from plants, animals, and the ocean. While all have their health benefits, each source has its limitations as the perfect omega-3 nutrient.

Omega-3s and Bioavailability

When we consume a food or drink, the nutrients contained are released, absorbed into the bloodstream, and transported to their respective target tissues. However, not all nutrients can be utilized to the same extent. In other words, they differ in their bioavailability and the way they are used in the human body.

Broadly defined, nutrient bioavailability refers to the fraction of a nutrient that is absorbed from the diet and made available for normal body functions. By definition, when a medication is administered intravenously, its bioavailability is 100 percent. It follows that for dietary supplements, herbs, and other nutrients, which are almost always taken orally, bioavailability will be much less.

The bioavailability of a nutrient is governed by multiple external and internal factors. External factors include the type of food and the chemical form of the nutrient in question. Gender, age, nutrient status, digestive enzymes, and life circumstance (pregnancy, for instance) are among the internal factors. The bioavailability of macronutrients (needed in large amounts), like carbohydrates, proteins, and fats, is usually greater than 90 percent of the amount ingested. But micronutrients (needed in trace amounts), like vitamins and minerals, can vary significantly in the extent to which they are absorbed and utilized.

Plant-Based Omega-3s

Alpha-linolenic acid is the primary omega-3 fat from plant-based sources, with the highest concentrations found in flaxseeds, chia seeds, and walnuts. Other rich sources of ALA include canola oil, soybeans, and leafy greens like kale and spinach. Lesser amounts are found in a variety of vegetables, including broccoli, Brussels sprouts, peas, and tomatoes.

Plant-based sources offer various health benefits mainly from the vitamins and other essential nutrients they contain, like magnesium; however, scientists believe their beneficial fat contribution is not impressive due to ALA's poor bioavailability. As described

When it comes to omega-3s, blood concentrations reflect both dietary intake and biological processes. The human body is able to utilize the long-chained EPAs and DHAs better than the short-chained ALAs. It is, however, able to synthesize (produce) EPAs and DHAs from ALAs—but only a small percentage. Because only a small amount is obtained this way, our bodies require direct intake of EPA and DHA.

The capacity to generate EPA and DHA from ALA is higher in women than men. Studies of ALA metabolism in healthy young men indicate that approximately 8 percent of dietary ALA is converted to EPA and zero to 4 percent is converted to DHA. In healthy young women, approximately 21 percent of dietary ALA is converted to EPA and 9 percent is converted to DHA. The better conversion efficiency of young women compared to men appears to be related to the effects of estrogen. In addition to gender differences, genetic variability in the enzymes involved in fatty acid metabolism influences one's ability to generate long-chain polyunsaturated fatty acids.

We, therefore, cannot rely on the consumption of ALAs alone to provide sufficient amounts of the other omega-3 fats. And don't assume that because you are taking a supplement that says it contains omega-3 fatty acids that your body is getting all that it needs. (More about this in "What About Fish Oil?," beginning on page 34.)

above in the inset "Omega-3s and Bioavailability," although the body is able to convert ALAs to the more bioavailable EPAs and DHAs, this conversion process is inefficient. You cannot rely on ALAs from food sources alone to provide an adequate amount of functional omega-3s. The consumption of fish, fish oil, and other marine-based sources like krill oil is necessary to maintain adequate levels.

Considerations

Along with the fact that plant-based omega-3s are only marginally effective, there are other issues to consider regarding the farming methods used for the plants themselves. It's no secret that the majority of farmers in the United States rely on the use of pesticides, insecticides, and herbicides to protect crops against insects and disease. It is also well known that these toxic chemicals have been linked to a wide range of human health problems, including various cancers, neurological damage, allergies, hormone disruption, and problems with reproduction and fetal development. Most herbicides, which are generally considered less toxic to animals and humans than insecticides, may interfere with a plant's hormones and enzymes, further altering its benefits to humans.

To avoid these harmful toxins, whenever possible, choose organically grown products. Not only does organically grown food taste better, it is also far more nutritious. Another reason organically grown food is recommended is that it means avoiding food that has been genetically modified.

Genetically modified (GM) food comes from *genetically modified organisms* (GMOs). Simply put, the genes of GM plants have been altered or artificially manipulated to mix and match the DNA of totally different species. Often this is done for the purpose of growing a bigger and supposedly better version of the crop. It is also done to create crops that are resistant to pesticides and herbicides. These crops can be doused with herbicide, which kills the weeds and pests but does not harm the crops themselves. Genetically modified corn, for example, may look picture perfect and even taste good, but think about what you are actually eating. A plant that is grown naturally would wither and die when doused with the same herbicide.

Concerns for the environment and human health are the most obvious reasons to avoid genetically modified foods. And people with food allergies need to be especially concerned as researchers are finding a growing number of links between the consumption of GM crops and the creation or worsening of allergies.

Organic foods are our best assurance against genetically modified organisms, which is why it is best to choose them whenever possible. But when it comes to omega-3s, plant-based sources in general are not sufficient for obtaining these beneficial fats.

Animal-Based Omega-3s

Arachidonic acid (AA), a fat from the omega-6 group, is found primarily in meats and other animal sources including milk and eggs. Some animals—primarily chickens and cows—that are fed (at least in part) a diet containing the plant-based omega-3s mentioned above, also supply omega-3s.

Like humans, when animals consume food containing alpha-linolenic acid (ALA), their bodies are able to convert a portion of it into EPA and DHA—the more bioavailable omega-3s. This means the meat and milk of pasture-raised cattle that feed largely on grasses and legumes contain boosted levels of these omega-3s (unlike most conventionally raised cattle that feed primarily on corn, which is high in omega-6s). Studies have also shown that meat from cattle that are fed grass-based diets have lower levels of two saturated fats that are known to increase harmful LDL blood cholesterol levels.

Eggs produced by chickens that are fed a diet of greens and flaxseeds, rather than corn, also contain higher levels of EPA and DHA. These levels are concentrated even further when the chickens are given fish oil and seaweed (algae).

While meat, eggs, and dairy products that contain increased levels of omega-3s may be better choices than those that do not, they should be consumed in moderation to avoid other possible health issues. Nutritionists have long warned that the saturated fat found in red meat raises LDL cholesterol and triglyceride levels.

Other Considerations

When it comes to animal-based omega-3s, it is important to consider the farming methods used for their feed. Are the plants they are fed grown organically—free of pesticides, herbicides, and chemicals from fertilizers? Are the sources GMO-free? Furthermore, many farm animals are given growth hormones, antibiotics, as well as a host of other "approved" chemicals. Adding to this concern are the many questionable additives put into processed meats, including (but not limited to) nitrates, monosodium glutamate (MSG), high levels of sodium, preservatives, and artificial coloring. This may be why study after study has shown that over-consumption of meat can increase the odds of getting cancer, as well as diabetes and heart disease.

Along with the negative health aspects of consuming meats, eggs, and other animal products, relying solely on them as good sources of omega-3s is not recommended. While certain products can offer boosted omega-3s, they are not sufficient.

Ocean-Based Omega-3s

The richest and most recommended sources of omega-3 fatty acids come from the sea—certain fish and other forms of marine life. But let's begin with their production on the first rung of the marine-life food chain—microalgae.

Omega-3s are formed in the chloroplasts of plankton (phyto-plankton, zooplankton)—a form of algae that is a food source for fish and other forms of sea life. Rich in EPA and DHA, these microalgae are also rich in astaxanthin—a powerful antioxidant that has been linked to numerous health benefits, including joint pain relief, healthy skin, and heart health.

Much like the grass-fed cattle mentioned earlier, many fish get their omega-3s from this "sea grass" (microalgae). These fish, as well as the fish that love to eat them, have the highest concentrations of DHA and EPA—the two healthiest forms of omega-3. Especially rich sources are Atlantic salmon and mackerel, cod, herring, bluefin tuna, sardines, and anchovies. Oils from these fatty fish have the best ratio of omega-3 to omega-6—about seven times more omega-3s than omega-6.

Fish are not able to produce these beneficial fats—they obtain them from eating plankton and other forms of microalgae, and store them as an energy source. It follows that fish whose diets consist predominantly of these omega-3-rich sea plants store the highest concentration of these fats in their tissues. If they live in a habitat where omega-3s are not widely available, they store much less. The close relationship between their diet and their omega-3 content applies to all of the specific omega-3s found in fish, including ALA, EPA, and DHA. It also applies to all types of fish, including wild-caught and farmed. Some farmed fish are fed processed omega-3 concentrates to boost their omega-3 content. Other farmed fish that are fed grains and soy meal have lower-than average omega-3 content. (See "Wild versus Farm-Raised Fish" on page 35.)

Considerations

Unfortunately, when it comes to eating fish as a rich source of omega-3s, you also need to take into the account the environment in which they live. When consuming fish (especially oily varieties) it is important to be aware of the potential presence of heavy metals and fat-soluble pollutants like polychlorinated biphenyls (PCBs) and dioxins, which contaminate ocean waters and accumulate in the aquatic food chain.

Smaller fish near the bottom of the food chain absorb mercury from water and aquatic plants. Because of their higher position, certain large predatory fish, particularly swordfish and sharks, absorb mercury from their prey and, in turn, contain high levels of mercury themselves. Mercury binds tightly to the proteins present in fish tissue, including muscle, and cooking does not reduce the mercury content. To illustrate further, let's say that throughout its lifespan, an anchovy eats sea plants that are contaminated with tiny amounts of mercury, which is present in the water. When a tuna comes along and eats many thousands of these anchovies over time, it is also absorbing the mercury they contain. The mercury then moves up the food chain even further as the contaminated tuna is consumed by larger fish, predatory birds, and humans.

Nearly all fish contain trace amounts of mercury, with shark, swordfish, king mackerel, ahi tuna, and tilefish having the highest levels due to their place near the top of the ocean food chain. According to the U.S. Environmental Protection Agency, salmon, sole, and anchovies are among those fish with the lowest levels.

Pregnant women need to be especially concerned with mercury because it can affect the development of their unborn child. For them, avoiding fish that are known to contain high mercury levels is strongly recommended, as is limiting the consumption of other fish. I have a number of patients who eat a lot of sushi and other kinds of fish. Through blood tests, I routinely check their mercury levels, which are often extremely high and explain their complaints of such nonspecific symptoms as fatigue, nausea, and muscle numbness and weakness. Cutting back on sushi and large amounts of fish almost always results in a resolution of symptoms. (If you eat a lot of fish, it is important to have your physician periodically check your mercury level.)

There is also concern that pesticide and herbicide use may have an effect on aquatic organisms. For example, the weed killer atrazine was found to have an adverse effect on frogs. This resulted in its ban in the European Union; however, atrazine remains one of the most widely used herbicides in the United States (over 70 million pounds per year). This and other such toxic products have been known to contaminate surface water and groundwater.

Although certain fish may be good sources of omega-3s, their possible health risks cannot be denied. You have to be careful when choosing your fish to minimize those that may contain higher levels of mercury in favor of species that contain less. I do recommend eating wild cold-water fish two to three times a week as part of healthy diet and as a way to obtain healthful omega-3s. However, because I am also concerned with the possible mercury content of fish, and knowing that most people don't eat enough fish to obtain sufficient amounts of EPA and DHA, I recommend supplementing with krill oil. I even recommend this supplement for people who eat fish occasionally.

Let me emphasize this point—I always prefer to obtain essential micronutrients from natural sources such as vegetables, fruits, nuts, legumes, and wild fish. But for most Americans who typically eat unhealthy diets, that is wishful thinking, and supplements are needed.

What About Fish Oil?

As you have just seen, when it comes to fish, there are a number of concerns regarding its status as a source of omega-3s. But what about fish oil supplements?

Wild versus Farm-Raised Fish

When comparing the omega-3 fat content of wild fish with that of farmed varieties, wild fish come out ahead. To explain why, it is important to consider what these fish eat. Wild seafood, whose diets consist largely of algae and other fish, are natural suppliers of EPA and DHA—the desirable long-chain omega-3s. On the other hand, conventional farm-raised fish—generally salmon, cod, sea bass, and catfish—are typically fed grains and soy meal, resulting in much smaller amounts of these healthful omega-3 fats. This type of feed does provide higher levels of ALA, which, unfortunately, is the less useful short-chain omega-3. (Some farmed fish are fed diets of fish meal and algae. They have higher omega-3 levels than conventionally farmed varieties.)

Along with being inferior suppliers of beneficial omega-3s, farmed fish have a number of other disadvantages. Because they are kept in cages, these fish have the tendency to be fattier, and have higher concentrations of omega-6 fats, which can cause inflammation in the body. As seen in the previous chapter, inflammation can lead to a number of serious health problems, including heart disease, arthritis, and asthma.

Again, depending on what they are fed, farmed fish can contain increased levels of organic toxins compared to wild-caught varieties. They have also been found to have greater concentrations of antibiotics and pesticides. This is because they are usually bred in a crowded environment, causing them to be more susceptible to disease. For this reason, farmers feed them antibiotics as a preventive. To combat sea lice—another common problem among farmed fish—they are also treated with pesticides.

Basically, not all fish are created equal. And fish, like people, are what they eat. Keep this in mind when comparing the omega-3 content of farmed fish with that of wild-caught. Also remember that even wild-caught fish—although richer sources of omega-3s than farmed—have a number of downsides.

Generally made from mackerel, herring, tuna, halibut, salmon, and cod liver, fish oil supplements—like the fish they come from—are rich sources of two omega-3 fatty acids, EPA and DHA.

Fish oil supplements have come under scrutiny in recent years as some brands were found to contain excessive levels of polychlorinated biphenyls. PCBs belong to a broad family of harmful organic chemicals called chlorinated hydrocarbons. They are found in hundreds of commercial products, including plastics, paints, rubber, dyes, and electrical and hydraulic equipment. When PCBs were found to cause cancer and other adverse health conditions, including compromised immune, reproductive, endocrine, and nervous systems, they were banned by the Environmental Protection Agency in 1979. They can, however, still be released into the environment from hazardous waste sites located near oceans, rivers, and streams. In the environment, PCBs are very stable compounds and do not decompose readily. They last for many years and are insoluble in water, which contributes to their stability. Their destruction by chemical, thermal, and biochemical processes is extremely challenging, which means they are difficult to eliminate from the environment as well as from the human body.

The majority of these questionable supplements came from the livers of cod and sharks. Unlike the oils processed from whole fish, these liver-based oils were believed to have a higher PCB content because of the liver's role as a major filtering and detoxifying organ. Even though the manufacture of PCBs was banned in 1979, low levels of this toxin are still present in some waters. In these waters, predatory fish at the top of the food chain, as well as bottom feeders, tend to contain the highest PCB levels.

Another very important omega-3 consideration is bioavailability. Once digested, the delivery of omega-3s to the bloodstream and eventual assimilation to target tissues depends on their form. The most common forms of omega-3 fats in marine oil supplements are triglycerides, ethyl esters, free fatty acids, and phospholipids.

The structure and breakdown of these forms are very different. This is relevant as it determines how much of the omega-3 capsule you swallow ends up arriving where you need it, in the joints, the brain, or the heart. A capsule that boasts a high amount of omega-3s isn't beneficial if only a small fraction actually survives digestion.

Of the available forms of omega-3s found in marine sources, recent studies have indicated that phospholipids are the most efficiently absorbed. Of the remaining forms, triglycerides circulate better than ethyl esters, while free fatty acids are 50 percent more efficient than triglycerides.

For the majority of fish oils sold globally, the EPA and DHA are in natural triglyceride form or ethyl ester form. Ethyl ester forms of fish oil are synthetically made by mixing free fatty acids with ethanol (alcohol). Omega-3 fish oils in the natural triglyceride form are preferable because they are more stable. This means they are less likely to form harmful oxidation products and are more bioavailable. What is ultimately important is to check the concentration of the forms of omega-3 in the fish oil brand you are considering. Those in ethyl ester form will be cheaper than those in triglyceride form, but the omega 3s will also be the least bioavailable, and therefore, the least useful to you.

In addition to fish oil's bioavailability, its digestibility is something else to consider—and not all forms are created equal. Many supplements cause gastrointestinal discomfort—indigestion, diarrhea, and those unpleasant burps that leave a fishy aftertaste. Also, depending on the dosage, large amounts can add needless calories to your diet.

Like fish, fish oil can be a rich source of omega-3s. While fish oil does offer certain health benefits, its status as the best source of omega-3s is questionable when considering bioavailability and digestibility. Fortunately there is an alternative to fish oil—krill oil. As you will see, supplemental krill oil is a purer, more bioavailable source of omega-3s than fish oil, and it has minimal if any side effects.

KRILL OIL

Nutrient-dense krill oil is extracted from tiny, bottom-of-the-food-chain shrimp-like crustaceans called krill, which are found in great abundance in the world's oceans. Researchers have found that the oil from krill provides superior omega-3 health benefits compared to fish oil. It is also purer and more bioavailable, making it a clear optimal choice.

Because of their place near the bottom of the ocean food chain, krill are considered the cleanest, purest source of omega-3s. They feed primarily on plankton—microscopic algae made up of tiny plants (phytoplankton) and animals (zooplankton)—which, as mentioned earlier in this chapter, is the first link in the food chain. Phytoplankton is rich in EPA and DHA. Whales, mantas, penguins, seals, and sharks are the primary consumers of krill.

Unlike most fish oil, in which the omega-3s are primarily in triglyceride form, those in krill oil are absorbed and carried to the body's cells in the form of phospholipids—the most effective carriers of EPA and DHA. This makes the fats in krill oil significantly more bioavailable than those in fish oil. As an added bonus, because it is more digestible, krill oil doesn't cause burping, reflux, or other discomforts associated with indigestion. The omega-3 phospholipids are also building blocks for cell membranes, red blood cells, brain cells, and joint tissue.

Another benefit of krill oil is that it contains *astaxanthin*—a strong antioxidant that protects cells, organs, and body tissues from oxidative damage. Responsible for the krill's red color (as well as the color of wild salmon and shrimp), astaxanthin is also a natural preservative that prevents the DHA and EPA in the oil from spoiling. Detailed information on krill and the benefits of krill oil, including why it is superior to fish oil, is discussed in Chapter 3.

CONCLUSION

Along with presenting the various sources of omega-3s, including their benefits and downsides, I have shown you why krill oil is a superior source. In the next chapter, you'll discover the science behind krill oil; how it was first discovered, tested, and introduced to the public; and why it is the best option for anyone who wants the purest, safest, most bioavailable source of omega-3s.

3

All About Krill

Named for the Norwegian word *kril,* which means "young fry of fish," krill are tiny ocean-dwelling crustaceans that play an integral role in the aquatic food chain. Not only are krill the primary diet for numerous fish and marine mammals, they are also the purest, most bioavailable source of omega-3 fatty acids—important nutrients for good health. Although you can't order a platter of krill at your local restaurant, fortunately, you are still able to obtain their omega fats through supplemental krill oil.

The story of krill's prominent place in the food chain is a fascinating one. That story and how krill relates to your health are subjects of this chapter, as is the science behind krill oil. You'll discover how something that is such a tiny part of the vast ocean can have such a dramatic impact on good health.

WHAT ARE KRILL?

Krill belong to the same crustacean family as shrimp, lobsters, and crabs. Though they average only about two inches in length, around the size of your pinky, as you will see, they represent a giant-sized link in the marine ecosystem. Shrimp-like in appearance, krill have large black eyes and a reddish, semi-transparent shell. Their segmented body has a soft chitin exoskeleton and many legs, which they use for swimming and eating. Sometimes called "the light-shrimp," krill periodically emit a yellow-green glow produced by bioluminescent organs located on their eye-stalks, hips, legs, and sternum. Scientists suggest this personal light show may play a part in their mating ritual as well as their night-time movement through the dark ocean waters.

There are about eighty-five species of krill with the Antarctic variety (*Euphausia superba*) as the largest and most dominant. They are also plentiful—with the total biomass in the Southern Ocean weighing an estimated 500 million tons. (This is roughly the esti-mated total weight of all humans on the earth.) With a lifespan of five to ten years, krill generally spend their days deep in the cold ocean waters. At night, when they are less likely to be spotted by whales, penguins, and sea birds—their major predators—they swim upward to feast on the omega-3-rich phytoplankton that is found near the ocean's surface. It is here in the icy waters sur-rounding Antarctica that one of the largest accumulations of phy-toplankton in the world exists. These deep waters are also considered most pristine with the lowest accumulation of toxins and other contaminants.

To confuse their predators, krill travel in swarms or "clouds" so they cannot be singled out. During certain times of the year, these swarms are so large and concentrated they can be spotted from space.

The main spawning season of the Antarctic krill is from Janu-ary to March. Females lay up to 10,000 eggs at once and can do so several times a season. Because the eggs are heavier than sea water, they sink to the ocean floor where they are safe enough to hatch. Then, in a process called *developmental ascent*, they make their way up through the ocean waters feeding on the yolk reserves as they mature. Females reach maturity in their third year; males mature in their fourth.

Along with phytoplankton, which is their primary food source, krill eat nutrient-rich detritus—organic material made of decomposing algae and sea organisms that drifts through the water as "marine snow." Depending on their developmental stage, they also consume the algae that grow on the underside of the pack ice. Krill can survive for long periods without food (up to two hundred days) and shrink in length as they starve.

Small krill are the main staple in the diets of literally hundreds of different fish and marine animals that live in the Antarctic. Without them, most of the marine life forms in the Antarctic would have evolved differently.

THE BENEFICIAL COMPONENTS OF KRILL

As you've seen, because of krill's placement on the bottom rung of the marine food chain and its life in the clean polar waters, the oil from this miniature crustacean is a nearly pure source of omega-3s—virtually free of toxins, metals, PCBs, dioxins, and other contaminants. Like krill oil, fish oil contains the beneficial long-chain omega-3s EPA and DHA; however, they differ in a number of ways. Three important advantages lie in the components of krill themselves—phospholipids, phosphatidyl-choline, and astaxanthin.

Phospholipids

As mentioned earlier in this chapter, the majority of the fatty acids EPA and DHA contained in krill oil are attached to phospholipids—a structure that makes them more absorbable than the triglyceride form, which is the structure found in most fish oils. This phospholipid structure allows for an easier entrance of the omega-3s into cells and facilitates a more efficient transfer to tissues such as the brain, liver, and kidneys.

Triglycerides are *hydrophobic*, which means they don't mix well with water. On the other hand, phospholipids are *amphipathic* and able to mix with both water and fats. This is important because it leads to better delivery and absorption of DHA and EPA in the body—making them significantly more bioavailable than those found in fish oil. In fact, recent studies have shown that krill oil is absorbed significantly better than fish oil.

A 2011 study determined the bioavailability of omega-3 fatty acids from three different sources: fish oil triglycerides, fish oil ethyl esters, and krill oil. Bioavailability of the EPA and DHA in krill oil was found to be highest of all sources, and 2.5 times better than fish oil. Scientific evidence to date maintains that phospholipids are the safest and most effective carriers of EPA and DHA—greatly facilitating the passage of the fatty acid molecules through the intestinal wall, and from there, directly into the tissues that need them.

Another benefit of krill oil over fish oil is that it is more easily digestible. About 80 to 85 percent of fish oil is never absorbed in the intestines, which causes about half of those who take it to experience burping and an unpleasant aftertaste. Conversely, the quick absorption of krill oil prevents these gastrointestinal side effects.

Phospholipids are superior to triglycerides not only because of better absorption, but also because they are metabolized and utilized better. For example, phospholipids follow simpler digestion and distribution routes, are components of cell membranes, are an important part of lipid transport as part of lipoproteins, cross the blood-brain barrier, and act as emulsifiers and carriers. In comparison, triglycerides are a source of stored energy in adipose (fatty) tissue, offer insulation and protection, and facilitate the transfer of fat-soluble vitamins.

Phosphatidyl-Choline

The phospholipids in krill have the added bonus of containing another essential nutrient, choline in the form of phosphatidyl-choline. To explain, the omega-3s in fish oil's triglyceride form are not able to be used by the body immediately. First, they must be attached to a molecule of phosphatidyl-choline (PC) by the liver. Only then is the body able to absorb them. Unlike fish oil, krill oil already contains the biologically active form of PC, so it can be absorbed by the body as is. It is quickly digested and then incorporated into the tissues of the brain, liver, and lungs.

Phosphatidyl-choline is composed partly of *choline*—the precursor of the vital neurotransmitter *acetylcholine*, which is responsible for sending nerve signals to the brain—and of *trimethylglycine,* which protects the liver. Choline is an important nutrient, important for a number of critical functions, including brain development, muscle control, learning, and memory. In fact, it plays a vital role in fetal and infant brain development, making it especially important for women who are pregnant or nursing. Usually grouped within the B-complex vitamins, choline is a recommended daily nutrient. The body can produce choline, but only in very small amounts—not enough to meet one's metabolic requirements. It is best obtained through foods or in a supplemental form. Krill oil contains this essential nutrient, which is another advantage over fish oil.

Astaxanthin

Another significant reason krill oil is superior to fish oil is that it is a rich source of astaxanthin—a powerful antioxidant that is effective in protecting phospholipid cell membranes from the damaging effects of harmful free radicals. Free radicals occur in everyday environments in the form of ultraviolet (UV) rays, rancid fats, and pollution, or as by-products in the body from breathing oxygen and digesting food for energy. By neutralizing free radicals, astaxanthin administers powerful protection for cells. It can help the skin block the sun's UV rays, but, fortunately, does not interfere with the formation of the essential nutrient vitamin D. Scientific evidence has shown repeatedly that antioxidants are key in the prevention of many diseases and health conditions, including cancer and heart disease. They also appear to play a role in slowing the aging process itself, including age-related mental decline.

A member of the carotenoid family, astaxanthin is red in color and naturally found in microalgae. When consumed, it is what gives certain sea creatures like shrimp and wild salmon their reddish-pink color (most farmed salmon get their color from artificial coloring). Krill, which serve as a natural food source for a number of ocean dwellers including salmon, contain astaxanthin in plentiful amounts. In krill oil's phospholipid form, a molecule of this beneficial antioxidant is attached to each EPA fatty acid.

Primarily due to its significant activity in fighting free radicals, astaxanthin has been linked to improved immune function and a number of other health benefits. Research is ongoing, and although further evidence is needed, early studies have suggested its positive effects in improving blood flow, reducing elevated triglyceride levels, and increasing beneficial HDL cholesterol. It has been used both topically and orally to promote healthy skin—helping to prevent dryness and wrinkles, and to reduce age spots. Study results have further suggested astaxanthin's possible role in reducing the symptoms of acid reflux, and in promoting heart health and general endurance. It has been used in the treatment of macular degeneration, Alzheimer's disease, and Parkinson's disease, and has been found to be effective in reducing cramps, bloating, mood swings, and other common menstrual and premenstrual discomforts.

Further studies are currently underway on astaxanthin's role in reducing the inflammation and joint pain associated with rheumatoid arthritis and carpal tunnel syndrome, as well as its effectiveness in treating certain cancers.

Another benefit of astaxanthin is that it is a natural preservative. Its presence in krill oil helps prevent the beneficial DHA and EPA fatty acids from oxidizing and becoming rancid. By comparison, fish oil, which does not contain astaxanthin, is highly perishable.

KRILL HARVESTING AND SUSTAINABILITY

At the beginning of krill fishery, krill was harvested largely as a food source for domesticated animals and even humans in certain countries like Japan and Russia. Over the past few decades, krill fishing, which occurs almost exclusively in Antarctic waters, has grown significantly and involves as few as five to eight countries. The miniature crustaceans are used primarily as feed for some farmed fish (particularly salmon, which get their pink color from the astaxanthin in krill), and mostly as bait for sports fishing in Japan and Korea. By the end of the 1990s, interest in krill expand-

From the Ocean to the Marketplace

The journey that lead to the discovery of krill oil as a superior omega-3 supplement began in the late 1990s. It was then that a team of researchers became interested in krill, the small, shrimplike crustaceans that live in the icy waters of the Southern Ocean and make up the central diet for whales, seals, penguins, and seabirds.

By 1998, a successful oil extraction method for krill was developed by Canadian-based Neptune Technologies & Bioressources. Soon after, one of Neptune's medical scientists, working with a team of chemists and engineers, discovered the oil's unique phospholipid molecular structure, which was different from the triglyceride structure of conventional fish oil. This turned out to be quite an important discovery.

The fact that krill oil's beneficial long-chain EPA and DHA fatty acids are carried on phospholipids is the primary reason for its advantage over other sources of these omega-3s. The researchers found that they are not only absorbed significantly better and faster than triglycerides, they are also used better by the human body. This is because phospholipids follow a much simpler digestion and distribution path leading to greater bioavailability, cellular absorption, and bioefficiency. Through continued research, the team also discovered that the oil contained astaxanthin—a powerful antioxidant that gives krill its beautiful red color.

What followed next was a series of studies to evaluate and confirm the safety and efficacy of this oil for human health. And in 2002, Neptune became the first company to bring supplemental krill oil to the marketplace. Today, more than a decade later, krill oil is recognized worldwide for its health benefits and superior absorption capabilities.

ed to the health industry when the precious omega-3 oils with phospholipids and the antioxidant astaxanthin they contain were first made available as a supplement. (See the inset on page 45.)

Following the slight rise of Antarctic krill harvesting, scientists and environmentalists began expressing concern over its sustainability. Krill feed on phytoplankton, and marine life feeds on krill. Without krill, a negative impact would ripple through the entire food chain. Realistically, this would seem to be an unlikely scenario due to krill's sheer volume, which, depending on the season, is estimated to be anywhere from 100 to 500 million tons. (Furthermore, its annual reproduction rate lies somewhere in the area of several hundred million tons.) However, in 1982, knowing the importance of krill in the Antarctic marine ecosystem, coupled with concern over increasing commercial interest, the Commission for the Conservation of Antarctic Marine Living Resources (CCAMLR) was established.

An international commission of members from twenty-five countries that make up several scientific committees, the CCAMLR is responsible for the preservation of marine ecosystems through research, eco-management, and conservation practices. By setting harvesting limits annually and monitoring commercial fishing activities in the Southern Ocean, the commission is able to ensure the sustainability of the krill supply. It has also begun identifying marine protected areas. To make sure CCAMLR's annual fishing regulations and quotas are being followed, two main independent organizations—Friends of the Sea (FOS) and the Marine Stewardship Council (MSC)—board the shipping vessels and audit them onsite.

The CCAMLR, to date, has not predicted a shortage of Antarctic krill, nor does it foresee a shortage in the near future. Keeping in mind that recent estimations of the krill biomass ranges from 100 to 500 million tons, and that current commercial harvesting is limited to 620,000 tons per year, this means that only a very small percentage (about 0.5 percent) of the total biomass is captured by fisheries.

What appears to be of greater concern to Antarctic krill is an environmental one. Scientists are becoming increasingly apprehensive that this network of life is being threatened by the climate change brought on by global warming. The western Antarctic Peninsula is warming at a fast rate. (It is, however, important to keep in mind that this peninsula is a northward-expanding appendix toward the southern tip of South America, and not representative of the entire Antarctic continent.) Winter temperatures have increased about 11°F over the past sixty years. One result of this warming trend is a reduction in the sea ice cover in that area (not the entire continent). How does this affect krill? For some time over its life cycle, krill feed on the microalgae that form on the underside of this polar ice, especially during their larval and juvenile stages. They also use the ice as a place to hide from predators.

Another climate change challenge for Antarctic krill, as well as many calcifying organisms, like coral, bivalve mussels, and snails, is the ocean's increasing levels of carbon dioxide (CO_2), which create a low pH environment. Krill's soft chitin exoskeleton contains carbonate, which is susceptible to dissolving in this environment (but not as susceptible as the shells of mollusks which are made of aragonite). Increased CO_2 can also disrupt the development of krill eggs and even prevent them from hatching. But this is an unlikely phenomenon, and one that, if actually occurred, wouldn't become a challenge for hundreds of years.

Solutions for these environmental issues have been the focus of scientists and researchers throughout the world. Hopefully, with continued efforts, an optimistic outcome to this threat to marine ecosystems will be reached.

On a positive note, under the watchful eye of the CCAMLR and with the responsible harvesting practices and eco-friendly techniques employed by commercial fisheries, krill can remain a sustainable global food source far into the future.

CONCLUSION

While both fish oil and krill oil are popular sources of omega-3 fatty acids, the information in this chapter has shown why krill oil is the superior choice. To summarize:

- The omega-3s in krill oil are in phospholipid form, making them more bioavailable than those in fish oil, which are in triglyceride form.

- Krill, whose placement is at the bottom of the food chain, are harvested from the deep pristine waters around Antarctica. The oil from this wild krill is pure, virtually free of environmental toxins. On the other hand, most fish oil is harvested from large predatory fish that live in contaminated waters and whose placement is near the top of the marine food chain.

- Krill oil is rich in astaxanthin—a potent antioxidant.

- Krill oil is more easily absorbed and digested than fish oil, eliminating any fishy burps or unpleasant aftertaste.

Now that you know the background of krill and the omega-3-rich oil they contain, it's time to take a closer look at krill oil's role in treating a number of specific health conditions.

4

Fighting Cardiovascular Disease

The leading cause of mortality in the United States, heart disease accounts for 25 percent of all recorded deaths. It strikes indiscriminately—teenagers and adults, men and women, blacks and whites—all are susceptible. It can kill quickly or it can linger for years, causing pain, depression, and a wide variety of painful and debilitating symptoms. Affecting over 80 million Americans today, heart disease is truly a modern-day plague.

Researchers have long believed that among the many benefits of omega-3 fatty acids is their ability to lower a number of important risk factors leading to cardiovascular disease. They reduce inflammation throughout the body, which can damage blood vessels. They have also been linked to decreasing unhealthy levels of triglycerides and LDL cholesterol, and are believed to play a role in lowering blood pressure and reducing the risk of stroke. Reducing blood clotting is also among the heart-healthy benefits of omega-3s.

As you already know, rich sources of these beneficial nutrients are fatty cold-water fish and the oil extracted from them. You also know that the discovery of krill as another rich source has led to supplemental krill oil as an even better choice. After presenting an overview of the most common cardiovascular diseases and conditions, this chapter focuses on the role of omega-3s in treating as well as the preventing this growing epidemic.

THE STATISTICS TELL A TALE

Consider these grim statistics from the American Heart Association's *Heart Disease and Stroke Statistics—2013 Update:*

- More than 2,150 Americans die of heart disease every day. That's an average of one death every thirty-nine seconds.

- An average of 150,000 Americans who die of heart disease each year are under 65 years of age, while 33 percent of all deaths caused by heart disease occur before the age of 75, which is well below the average life expectancy of 77.9 years.

- Coronary heart disease causes one out of every six deaths in the United States each year, while one out of every eighteen deaths is caused by stroke.

- An average of 800,000 Americans die of heart disease each year.

- Each year, an estimated 785,000 Americans have a heart attack, and 470,000 more have a repeat attack.

- Approximately 195,000 Americans experience their first silent (unnoticed or undiagnosed) heart attack each year.

- About every twenty-five seconds, an American will have a coronary event; and about every minute, someone will die from one.

Although mortality rates caused by heart disease have started to decline over the past fifty years, the overall toll continues to rise, both in terms of impaired health and financial cost.

Here is the most important statistic to remember: For half of the people who die of a heart attack, death is the first and last heart-related symptom that they ever experience. In other words, prior to their deaths, most victims never experienced any sort of symptom to warn them that they were at risk for a heart attack. This is why it is so important to regularly work with your physician to determine your risk and monitor the health of your heart and overall cardiovascular system.

THE MOST COMMON TYPES
OF CARDIOVASCULAR DISEASE

After looking at the sobering statistics above, the devastation caused by cardiovascular disease is certainly obvious. Before discussing the positive effects of omega-3 fatty acids on these conditions, let's take a closer look at the most common heart problems —their classic symptoms, causes, and risk factors. Diagnosis and treatment of these problems will vary, and—like all matters involving your physical health—should be supervised under the watchful eye of a doctor or other healthcare professional.

Angina Pectoris

Derived from the Latin term for "squeezing of the chest," *angina pectoris* is chest pain caused by a decreased supply of blood to the heart muscle, usually due to a lesion on the walls or valves of the heart, or because of a narrowing of the coronary arteries. As a result of this constriction or blockage, the heart receives less oxygen—a condition called *ischemia*.

Risk factors for angina pectoris include smoking, lack of exercise, chronic stress, and high blood pressure. Being overweight or obese also increases risk, as does diabetes. The risk for angina also increases with age.

Typical symptoms of angina include pain, pressure, or other discomfort in the middle of the chest. This chest pain can radiate to the throat, jaw, upper back, arms, and even teeth. Unfortunately, cases of angina often go misdiagnosed or undiagnosed in women, who are more likely to suffer atypical symptoms, including palpitations, dizziness, heartburn, indigestion, nausea, numbness in the arms, weakness, and/or shortness of breath.

There are two types of angina: stable and unstable. *Stable angina* is the most common type, and is characterized by typical symptoms that are predictable. Ordinarily, symptoms last for around five minutes or so, and then begin to subside. *Unstable angina* is a more serious condition, with symptoms being more severe and less predictable, and usually lasting much longer.

Because this type of angina is often a precursor to and warning sign of a heart attack, prompt medical attention should be sought at the first sign.

It is essential that all angina sufferers make certain lifestyle changes to lower their risk of heart attack. This would include following a heart-friendly diet, maintaining a healthy weight, exercising regularly, reducing stress, and maintaining appropriate levels of cholesterol and blood sugar.

Atherosclerosis

Atherosclerosis refers to a hardening or blockage of the arteries due to the accumulation of a waxy substance called plaque. Plaque builds up as part of your body's inflammatory response to damage in artery walls. When arteries are damaged as the result of inflammation caused by high blood pressure, cigarette smoke, environmental toxins, or the presence of other irritants, your body sends cholesterol and other substances to the wound in an attempt to repair it. Collectively, these fatty deposits are known as plaque; over time, they can build up, narrowing and hardening the arteries. This, in turn, reduces blood flow and increases blood pressure levels.

Risk factors for atherosclerosis include age, diabetes and insulin resistance, high blood pressure, high cholesterol, obesity, smoking, and a family history of heart disease. Inflammation is an integral part of the process by which atherosclerosis develops.

Symptoms of atherosclerosis depend on the extent of the blockage and the specific arteries affected. In arteries of the heart, atherosclerosis can manifest as chest pain or pressure (angina), while in the arteries of the leg or arm, it can cause intermittent pain. In the arteries leading to the brain, atherosclerosis can produce warning signs of stroke, including slurred speech, drooping facial muscles, and numbness or weakness in the arms or legs. In arteries leading to the genitals, atherosclerosis can cause erectile dysfunction in men; while in women, the same condition can reduce blood flow to the vagina, resulting in less pleasurable sex. Unfortunately, many patients will not show symptoms until the atherosclerosis is severe, blocking over 70 percent of the affected artery, making this condition more difficult to diagnose and treat.

Should atherosclerosis be detected, your doctor may prescribe aspirin or cholesterol-lowering drugs or natural alternatives. You will probably be asked to make certain lifestyle changes, involving a low-cholesterol diet, regular exercise, and the avoidance of unhealthy behaviors such as smoking and alcohol consumption. Because stress is a major risk factor for heart disease, learning to reduce or control it is essential for the proper treatment of atherosclerosis. Adopting these lifestyle changes can prevent plaque from developing or progressing, significantly reducing the risk of atherosclerosis from developing.

Cardiac Arrest

Cardiac arrest, also known as *cardiopulmonary* or *circulatory arrest, sudden cardiac arrest,* and *sudden cardiac death,* is a condition in which the heart abruptly stops beating. This differs from heart attack in that the disruption of blood flow is not caused by a physical blockage, but rather by an electrical disturbance that impairs the heart's ability to pump blood to the rest of the body. And while the heart may continue to beat during a heart attack, it stops completely in cardiac arrest. As a result, blood ceases to flow, preventing oxygen from being delivered to the body and brain. Cardiac arrest is a very serious medical emergency. The majority of cases that are not treated within ten minutes end in death; those who survive are likely to suffer brain damage due to the loss of blood flow and needed oxygen to the brain.

The immediate cause of cardiac arrest is usually a severe arrhythmia such as ventricular fibrillation, in which the heartbeat cycle is electrically disrupted to the point of stopping altogether. But this life-threatening arrhythmia is itself the result of an underlying heart condition, usually coronary artery disease, although occasionally an enlarged and weakened heart (cardiomyopathy), heart valve disease, or congenital heart defect is to blame. Cardiac arrest can also be caused by noncardiovascular sources, including trauma, gastrointestinal bleeding, or hemorrhaging inside the cranium. Other factors that compound the risk of cardiac arrest include age (this increases in men over forty-five and women over fifty-five), smoking, high blood pressure, being overweight or obese, lack of exercise, diabetes, excessive alcohol consumption, drug use, and a previous history of heart disease. Men's risk for cardiac arrest is two to three times greater than that of women, and blacks are about one-third as likely as other groups to survive.

Symptoms of cardiac arrest appear suddenly and must be treated immediately. A victim of cardiac arrest will collapse, unconscious, unable to breathe, and with no pulse. Sometimes the arrest is preceded by a period of faintness or dizziness, chest pains, shortness of breath, nausea, or vomiting. These symptoms must be taken seriously. Contact 911 as immediate treatment is crucial for survival.

Because cardiac arrest is frequently fatal, prevention is often the best cure. If you are at risk, your doctor may advise you to make lifestyle changes. Don't smoke, drink moderately or not at all, eat a balanced diet, and get plenty of exercise; these choices will improve your health and help lower your vulnerability to cardiac arrest.

Congestive Heart Failure

Congestive heart failure (CHF) is a condition in which the heart is unable to pump a sufficient supply of blood to the rest of the body. CHF can be either chronic and ongoing or sudden and acute. Most cases of CHF initially develop in the heart's main blood pumping chamber, the left ventricle. CHF gets its name because when it occurs, blood backs up into, or congests, the liver, abdomen, lungs, and/or legs, ankles, and feet. Left untreated, CHF can cause heart valve problems, heart attack, stroke, and damage to the liver and kidneys.

CHF can be caused by a variety of conditions that weaken or damage the heart, including coronary heart disease, heart attack, high blood pressure, congenital heart defects, damaged heart muscle or valves, inflammation of the heart, arrhythmia, and atherosclerosis. Risk for CHF can be increased by various non-cardiovascular diseases, including severe anemia, diabetes and certain diabetes medications, hyperthyroidism and hypothyroidism, emphysema, lupus, infections, kidney disease, blood clots in the lungs, smoking, and excessive alcohol consumption.

There are many symptoms of CHF, ranging from chest pain and shortness of breath (after exertion or when lying down), fatigue, weakness, edema (swelling in ankles, feet, or legs), rapid or irregular heartbeat, swelling in the abdomen, sudden weight gain due to fluid retention, and nausea. All of these symptoms are typically more severe in cases of sudden CHF.

Patients with CHF are often advised to weigh themselves each morning and to notify their doctors if they experience a weight gain of three pounds or more over a twenty-four hour period. Such weight gain is usually a sign of fluid retention, indicating the need for adjusted treatment. CHF patients are also advised to achieve and maintain a healthy weight, to follow a low-fat, low-salt diet, and to limit their intake of alcohol and, in more severe cases, other fluids.

Coronary Heart Disease

Coronary heart disease (CHD), also called *coronary artery disease,* is a type of atherosclerosis that occurs specifically in the arteries of the heart. Once the inner wall of a coronary artery becomes diseased or damaged, fatty deposits composed of cholesterol and other cellular waste products—plaque—accumulate in the coronary artery walls, hardening and narrowing these vessels and restricting blood flow. Because the coronary arteries are already narrower than your other arteries, the effects of this particular type of atherosclerosis can be serious: deprived of blood, your heart can simply stop working.

As with atherosclerosis, CHD can be caused by a variety of factors, including poor diet and lack of exercise, high blood pressure, smoking, chronic stress, high levels of harmful LDL cholesterol and low levels of beneficial HDL cholesterol, and other health conditions, including diabetes, sleep apnea, and obesity. Radiation therapy, especially when used to treat certain cancers, can also cause CHD.

Initially, symptoms of CHD may not be apparent, but as the condition worsens, so, too, do the symptoms. As the artery blockages grow, CHD can manifest as angina (chest pain), and shortness of breath. Left untreated, CHD can result in arrhythmia, heart muscle failure, heart attack, or sudden death.

Because CHD is a "silent" killer—meaning you can suffer from the disease without experiencing any of its symptoms—regular medical checkups are important for everyone, but especially those who are considered to have a higher risk for developing this serious disease.

Heart Attack (Acute Myocardial Infarction)

A heart attack, or acute myocardial infarction (AMI), occurs when blood flow to the heart is interrupted, causing heart muscle cells to die. Lack of blood flow to the heart is most often due to a blockage of a coronary artery caused by vulnerable plaque—an unstable combination of cholesterol, fatty acids, and white blood cells that can form on the arterial wall in response to inflammation. When vulnerable plaque ruptures, blood clots can form, blocking the artery and diminishing blood flow, thus reducing oxygen supply to the heart and causing damage or death to heart muscle cells and tissues. The result is often fatal.

A wide range of factors can increase the risk of heart attack, including age, poor diet, lack of exercise, smoking, diabetes, being overweight or obese, chronic stress, high levels of physical exertion, high blood pressure, excessive alcohol consumption, the overuse of pharmaceutical or illegal drugs, kidney disease, and a personal or family history of heart disease.

Symptoms of AMI may be "silent," meaning they may occur without being noticed. When symptoms are apparent, they occur gradually, over the course of several minutes. The most common symptoms of AMI are chest pain (which can spread down the left arm and/or the left side of the neck), shortness of breath, nausea, vomiting, excessive sweating, and chest palpitations. In women, symptoms may not be as intense or as varied, and most commonly manifest as shortness of breath, fatigue, weakness, and sensations similar to indigestion. In the most serious cases, loss of consciousness or sudden death can also occur.

AMI patients are usually prescribed various heart medications, and are typically advised to make necessary dietary and lifestyle changes; stress management can be the key to a successful recovery.

High Blood Pressure (Hypertension)

High blood pressure, or hypertension, affects 76.4 million Americans today. Blood pressure is essentially a measure of the force (pressure) exerted by circulating blood on the walls of your arteries. Hypertension occurs when the force becomes so strong that it begins to stretch or cause damage to the arteries. Serious cases of hypertension can eventually create other health problems, including heart attack and stroke.

There are two types of hypertension: primary (essential) hypertension and secondary hypertension. *Primary hypertension* usually develops gradually over many years, and can be caused by a number of genetic and environmental factors, including age, gender, race, family history, stress, excessive sodium or alcohol consumption, poor diet, lack of exercise, and being overweight or obese. *Secondary hypertension* is usually caused by an underlying health condition, such as kidney disease, adrenal gland tumors, congenital heart conditions, or by the use of pharmaceutical drugs, including birth control pills, cold and flu remedies, decongestants, and pain medications. Illegal drugs, such as amphetamines and cocaine, are other possible causes.

Most of the time, there are no symptoms of hypertension. When they do appear—the most common being dull headaches, dizzy spells, and nose bleeds—it is usually a sign that the condition has progressed.

Proper treatment of hypertension begins with a healthy, low-sodium diet, regular moderate exercise, and stress management. Blood pressure medications may also be necessary. Once diagnosed, regular checkups are important to monitor the condition.

Stroke

A stroke is caused when the blood supply to the brain is interrupted or severely reduced, either because an artery has ruptured (burst) or because it has been blocked by a clot. Deprived of oxygen and other nutrients that the blood transports, brain cells begin to die within minutes after a stroke occurs. Prompt medical attention is, therefore, essential to limiting brain damage and other potential complications. Nearly 800,000 Americans will experience a stroke each year; it is the fourth most common cause of death in the United States and a leading cause of disability.

There are two main types of stroke: ischemic and hemorrhagic. *Ischemic stroke* is the more common and accounts for 87 percent of all strokes. It occurs when an artery to the brain becomes blocked by a blood clot, causing severely reduced blood flow (ischemia). There are two subcategories of ischemic strokes: *thrombotic strokes,* in which the blood clot forms in an artery that has already been narrowed (usually by atherosclerosis), and *embolic strokes,* in which the clot breaks off from another location (usually the heart) and travels to one of the brain's blood vessels, which are too narrow to allow the clot through.

Hemorrhagic stroke is caused by a blood vessel that ruptures and then leaks blood into the brain. There are two subcategories of hemorrhagic stroke. The first is the *intracerebral hemorrhage,* in which a blood vessel in the brain bursts, spilling its contents into surrounding brain tissue, damaging brain cells and depriving them of oxygen. The second type is the *subarachnoid hemorrhage,* which is caused by the bursting of an artery or aneurysm (abnormal bulge or "balloon" in a blood vessel) on or near the surface of the brain.

A variety of factors increase the risk of stroke, including poor nutrition and diet, hypertension, lack of regular physical activity, being overweight or obese, smoking or regular exposure to secondhand smoke, diabetes, a previous history of heart disease, excessive alcohol consumption, the use of illegal drugs such as cocaine and amphetamines, and sleep apnea, a condition in which oxygen levels fluctuate and drop during the night due to intermittent interrupted breathing. Use of birth control pills can also increase the risk of developing blood clots, and, thus, stroke. In addition, race can be a factor; statistically, African Americans have a higher risk for stroke than whites and other groups.

Symptoms vary according to the type and severity of the stroke. They include sudden dizzy spells, loss of coordination or difficulty walking, slurred speech, difficulty understanding speech, blurred or blackened vision in one or both eyes, paralysis or numbness of the face, arm or leg. A person who suffers a hemorrhagic stroke may also experience a sudden, sharp headache, which may or may not be accompanied by vomiting. At the first sign of symptoms, dial 911 for immediate medical attention, for the sooner you receive treatment, the higher your chances will be for a successful recovery.

THE RISK FACTORS

The best way to manage cardiovascular disease is to prevent it from happening in the first place. In addition to regular screenings from your doctor, true prevention involves addressing the known risk factors. Each of the diseases and conditions just discussed share many of the same common risks, which include one or more of the following:

- Obesity or being significantly overweight

- High blood pressure (hypertension)

- High LDL and total cholesterol levels

- Low HDL cholesterol levels

- Lack of exercise

- Poor diet

- Smoking

- Stress and uncontrolled emotions

- Type 2 (adult-onset) diabetes and prediabetes

Risk factors fall into two categories: uncontrollable and controllable. As the name implies, uncontrollable risk factors are those over which we have no control, such as age, hereditary (your genes), and family history of heart disease.

By contrast, controllable risk factors are those we *can* manage. Although doing so does not guarantee that you will never develop heart disease, at the very least, proactive behavior allows you to improve your mindset and your health in other areas.

THE CURRENT VIEW OF HEART DISEASE

When doctors and scientists talk about the causes of heart disease, they are often referring to the development of atherosclerosis, which, as you have just seen, is a condition in which the arteries become narrowed or hardened due to the buildup of a fatty substance called plaque. Because atherosclerosis sets the stage for the development of many serious heart conditions, including heart attack, angina, and stroke, its prevention is vital. Find the cause of atherosclerosis, and you will find the cause of many of the most common forms of heart disease. Find the cure for atherosclerosis and you will save millions of lives—and get a Nobel Prize!

How Does Heart Disease Develop?

Over the last twenty years, the medical community has come to believe that the root cause of atherosclerosis—and, thus, much heart disease—is chronic inflammation. This idea was first formally introduced in the mid-1990s by then-president of the American Heart Association, Valentin Fuster, and further refined a decade later by Peter Libby, the director of the Donald W. Reynolds Cardiovascular Clinical Research Center at Harvard University. According to Fuster and Libby, inflammation is the mechanism that drives the development of both atherosclerotic (hard) plaque and vulnerable (soft) plaque—an unstable material that can easily rupture, sending clots into the bloodstream, where they can block arteries and cause heart attack or stroke.

To understand Fuster and Libby's theory of how heart disease works, we first need to look at the concept of inflammation. As I mentioned in Chapter 1, inflammation is essentially an immune response—your body's way of coping with an injury or threat to its well-being. Remember, there are two types of inflammation: acute and chronic. Acute (short-term) inflammation occurs in response to a bodily insult: a cut, an infection, a burn, or other physical injury. Within seconds of cutting your finger, for example, your body's immune response kicks in, sending blood cells, proteins, and other healing compounds to the affected area and begins the healing process. Your finger turns red, bleeds, and swells as blood rushes to the area. Eventually, the blood clots around the cut, and the redness and swelling reduces as the healing process advances. That is your body's immediate "acute inflammation" response at work.

Chronic (long-term) inflammation occurs when an acute inflammation response fails to heal or resolve an injury, or in response to prolonged exposure to a stressor. Sometimes chronic inflammation can even occur in the absence of any harmful or invasive agent. As your body tries to heal itself without success, the types of cells that are present at the site of the injury start to change, potentially causing extensive damage to both healthy and the already-impaired tissue. Because it often affects internal organs, chronic inflammation usually lacks the obvious symptoms that characterize acute inflammation, and can be difficult to diagnose. Its effects, however, are quite powerful. Because of the progressive damage it inflicts on your tissues, chronic inflammation has been linked to a number of serious health conditions, including arthritis, asthma, gastrointestinal disorders, cancer, and heart disease.

According to the inflammation model of heart disease, when an artery is torn, ruptured, or otherwise damaged by infection, high blood pressure, cigarette smoke, or other offending factors, your body initiates an inflammatory response, ordering cholesterol, blood cells, clotting proteins, minerals, and other agents to the site of the damage in order to protect and heal it. These agents embed in the wall of the artery and slowly accumulate, forming a pliable substance called soft plaque, whose outer surface is covered by a fibrous cap. Unfortunately, sometimes this cap is very thin, making the plaque unstable, easily damaged, and prone to rupture. This soft plaque is considered vulnerable because it is so weak.

After time, the body begins to treat this vulnerable plaque as a new invader, essentially instigating an inflammatory cascade, or an inflammatory response to the original inflammatory response. In this new inflammatory response, fresh blood cells, cholesterol, minerals, and other healing agents are sent to fight the plaque. There are two possible outcomes to this event. When attacked by these blood cells, the fibrous cap that covers vulnerable plaque can rupture, spilling the powerful coagulants found in its interior into the bloodstream, where they thicken the blood and can form large and lethal clots. Left untreated, these clots can block the arteries—a condition called *thrombosis,* which can ultimately lead to heart attack or stroke.

Alternatively, the calcium and other minerals sent to the plaque can help stabilize it, adhering to the plaque's sticky surface and solidifying its fibrous cap. At first glance, this inflammatory response—an attempt to protect your body against further damage—might seem like a good thing since the plaque can no longer rupture. But in fact, this outcome is still troublesome, since the plaque is now there to stay, building up within the artery walls and causing them to harden and narrow. In short, as a result of the inflammatory cascade (repeated inflammatory response), atherosclerosis develops—opening up new risks for a host of other cardiovascular conditions, including heart attack, stroke, angina, and more.

How is Heart Disease Treated?

Knowing what they know, how do doctors then decide to treat heart disease? Because scientific understanding of inflammation is still developing, physicians in the United States treat and prevent heart disease in part by attempting to control the risk factors that seem to contribute to its development, like high LDL cholesterol or triglycerides, and low HDL cholesterol. Many of these risk factors can be reduced or removed by adopting lifestyle changes—

quitting smoking, eating a more wholesome diet, becoming more physically active, maintaining a proper weight, and eliminating or limiting stressors. In addition, doctors often prescribe drugs to help control these risk factors, including aspirin to thin the blood and angiotensin-converting enzyme (ACE) inhibitors and beta blockers to lower blood pressure.

The risk factor that doctors most frequently focus on and treat through medication is high cholesterol. Large-scale research studies consistently identify cholesterol as one of the prime culprits in raising the likelihood of heart disease. As a result, doctors often try to lower cholesterol in their patients by prescribing a class of drugs called statins. Statins do work—but not for everyone. Studies reliably show that statins either reduce or prevent the recurrence of coronary events (heart attacks, strokes, etc.) in patients who have already experienced one.

The problem with statins is that they are overwhelmingly prescribed for patients who have high cholesterol levels but who have never experienced a cardiac event. In an important review of eleven of the largest-scale studies investigating the use of statins, with a combined data pool of over 65,000 subjects, a recent report published in the *Journal of the American Medical Association* found that there was no evidence that statins had any benefits for heart disease prevention in patients who had never before been diagnosed with a cardiovascular condition. That is to say, if you've never experienced a heart attack, stroke, or other heart condition, statins are unlikely to prevent those coronary events from occurring—even if your risk for heart disease is high! Statins simply will not help people who don't already have cardiovascular disease. If anything, they can do more harm than good for these people, who may suffer unnecessary and unpleasant side effects without proof of benefit.

BENEFITS OF OMEGA-3s AND KRILL OIL

The old adage that "prevention is the best medicine" is good, solid advice, and being proactive is the best approach for dealing with any health condition. When it comes to lowering your risk of cardiovascular disease, there are many aspects of your life that you can control. Making sure your diet includes the right omega-3 fatty acids is one of them. When looking to give your heart health a boost, there is plenty of evidence that omega-3s play an important role in improving cardiovascular health and decreasing the risk of developing heart disease.

In Chapter 1, you saw that among the benefits of omega-3 fats (primarily EPA and DHA) is their effectiveness in reducing unhealthy levels of triglycerides and LDL cholesterol. They also tend to lower blood pressure. Further, they can help prevent and treat atherosclerosis by slowing the development of artery-clogging plaque and blood clots.

Fish and fish oil have long been known as a rich source of the omega-3 fats EPA and DHA. For this reason, much of the existing research on the benefits of these fats has come from studies involving these sources. So far, the results have been impressive:

- The GISSI-Prevenzione Trial of 11,324 heart attack survivors showed that dietary supplementation of low-dose fish oil significantly reduced their risk of having another heart attack or stroke.

- Danish researchers concluded that fish oil supplementation may help prevent arrhythmias (irregular heartbeat) and sudden cardiac death in healthy men.

- American medical researchers reported that men who consumed fish once or more every week have a 50-percent lower risk of dying from a sudden cardiac event than men who eat fish less than once a month.

Let's take a closer look at some of the more important studies on fish oil. The first major study to evaluate the effects of fish oil on heart disease was the Diet and Reinfarction Trial (DART), which began in the United Kingdom in 1983. Over two years, the DART researchers followed 2,033 men who had recently recovered from a heart attack. A third of the subjects were assigned a lower-fat diet with a high ratio of polyunsaturated to saturated fat, a third of the subjects were assigned a diet high in cereal fiber

(fiber found in whole grains), and a third of the subjects were told to eat at least two portions of fish or the equivalent in fish oil supplements each week. Initially, the scientists believed that the group with the lower-fat diet would see the greatest health improvements. So they were incredibly surprised to find that it was the fish- and fish-oil-eating group that actually came out ahead. When compared to the people in the other two groups, members of the fish-eating group were significantly less likely to die—not only from coronary heart disease, but from all other serious conditions not related to heart disease. Their death rates from all causes of mortality were 29 percent lower than those seen in the other two groups. Statistically speaking, that's a huge reduction in mortality! The results were intriguing, suggesting that fish oil could help protect the hearts of people who were already suffering from cardiovascular disease, allowing them to live longer.

The DART study paved the way for more extensive investigation into the use of fish oil in preventing heart disease, especially in those with risk factors. In the Japan EPA Lipid Intervention Study (JELIS), scientists conducted a trial with over 18,000 middle-aged and older subjects, all of whom had high total cholesterol levels. Both groups were prescribed statin drugs, but half the subjects were also given an additional supplement of 1.8 grams of EPA that had been derived from fish oil. While both groups experienced a decrease in their total cholesterol, LDL cholesterol, and triglyceride levels, the change was greater in the group that had been given the fish oil supplements. More important, over the course of the four-and-a-half-year study, subjects who had taken the supplements were found to have experienced significantly fewer major coronary events (sudden cardiac death, heart attack, unstable angina, and heart surgeries)—19 percent less than the group that had only taken the statins. While this study doesn't measure the efficacy of fish oil as a standalone measure for preventing heart disease, it indicates that fish oil may be a potent addition to a preventive regimen.

Similarly, in the Nurses' Health Study, a large-scale study of 84,688 female nurses conducted over a period of sixteen years, researchers found that women who ate fish more than once a month had a lower risk of coronary heart disease than did women who rarely or never ate fish. Moreover, the women who regularly ate fish were also less likely to die from coronary heart disease than were their non-fish-eating counterparts. And the more fish the women ate, the more they reduced their risk of dying from coronary heart disease. Women who ate fish one to three times each month lowered their risk by 21 percent, women who ate fish once a week lowered their risk by 29 percent, women who ate fish two to four times a week lowered their risk by 31 percent, and women who ate fish five or more times a week lowered their risk by 34 percent.

Preliminary evidence suggests that the high levels of omega-3 fatty acids found in fish oil are particularly effective at lowering triglyceride levels. By some estimates, regular consumption of fish oil supplements can reduce triglycerides by 25 to 30 percent. Fish oil also seems to help reduce the inflammation that serves as a major risk factor for heart disease. In a study published in the journal *Atherosclerosis,* test subjects who were given a combination of fish oil and plant sterols (a natural oil found in plants) saw significant reductions in their levels of inflammation. Blood levels of hs-CRP—an important biomarker, or measurable indicator, of inflammation—dropped by an average of 39 percent. Looking at this dramatic decline in inflammation, the researchers estimated that supplementing with fish oil and plant sterols could reduce the overall risk of cardiovascular disease by almost 23 percent.

In an analysis of sixty-eight different studies on fish oil, Chinese researchers also concluded that fish oil had "a significant lowering effect" on several key markers of inflammation, including C-reactive protein (CRP) and interleukin-6 (IL-6). What's more, the effect occurred not only in healthy individuals, but also in subjects who either had or were at high risk of developing heart disease. This suggests that fish oil may not only help prevent heart disease, but may also potentially keep the disease from progressing further in those who already have it.

How do studies on fish and fish oil relate to krill oil? Like fish oil, krill oil is a rich source of the omega-3 fats said to be responsible for improving heart health. Accordingly, many of the cardiovascular benefits of fish oil can be attributed to krill oil as well. Research generally confirms that the two oils are at least comparable in terms of quality. In fact, some early studies suggest that when it comes to protecting your heart, krill oil may be an even better option than fish oil. As I've explained, krill oil's unique phospholipid form increases the bioavailability of the EPA and DHA contained within, giving your body easier access to these fats and allowing them to be used much more readily.

Research over the past few years supports this idea. In a study published in the 2013 issue of the *Lipids in Health and Disease,* scientists compared the capacities of both krill oil and fish oil in increasing blood levels of EPA, DHA, and total long-chain n-3 PUFAs. The researchers found that the EPA and DHA were significantly better absorbed when taken in krill oil than fish oil. Furthermore, it is important to note that krill oil reduced omega-6 fatty acids significantly more as compared to fish oil. As previously described, too much omega-6 may promote inflammation.

A number of studies have found krill oil to be much more effective than fish oil at reducing blood levels of triglycerides, total cholesterol, and LDL cholesterol. It was also more effective at lowering blood glucose levels. As you'll recall, better glucose control is integral to lowering the risk of insulin resistance and diabetes, two conditions that can contribute to the risk of cardiovascular disease. In one study, researchers compared the effects of krill oil and fish oil on lipid levels. They found that patients who took 3 grams of krill oil each day saw their total cholesterol levels decline by 18 percent, their LDL cholesterol levels decline by 39 percent, and their triglyceride levels decline by 27 percent. Meanwhile, the krill-taking group also saw HDL cholesterol levels rise by a whopping 60 percent. In comparison, patients who took 3 grams of fish oil saw their total cholesterol decrease by only 6 percent, their LDL cholesterol by 5 percent, and their triglyceride levels decline by 3 percent. HDL levels increased by a mere 4 percent. What's more, the researchers found that taking just 1.5 grams of krill oil was significantly more effective in lowering LDL cholesterol and glucose than taking twice that amount (or 3 g) of fish oil. Clearly, krill oil's potential is undeniable.

There's some evidence that krill oil may even offset some of the risk factors for cardiovascular disease. One animal study also indicated that krill oil lowered total cholesterol and glucose levels not only in rats who were fed the equivalent of a balanced diet, but also in rats who consumed a diet high in fat. This suggests that krill oil may help compensate for a less-than-optimal diet or body mass index, although obviously it is not meant to be a substitute for improving a person's lifestyle choices.

Another animal study suggests that krill oil may play a role not only in lowering the risk of heart disease, but in directly protecting the heart itself. Rats who were given regular doses of krill oil saw their total and LDL cholesterol decrease in comparison to rats who received no krill oil. More important, after heart attacks were induced in all the rats, those who had received the krill oil experienced a lesser degree of cardiac hypertrophy, a condition in which the heart muscle tissue thickens and enlarges. This is important because cardiac hypertrophy prevents the heart from pumping as forcefully as it might under healthier circumstances, increasing the risk of heart failure, heart attack, and stroke.

The rise of scientific interest in the benefits of krill oil on cardiovascular health has resulted in a growing number of clinical studies (both animal and human) on the potential of this valuable supplement. I look forward to the discovery of an even greater number of positive results in the near future.

CONCLUSION

Because krill oil is a relatively new product, research on its cardiovascular benefits is still in its infancy. It will take some time before scientists understand the full range of its health advantages. But the early results are promising, indicating that krill oil may be a better omega-3 source than fish oil when it comes to helping prevent and possibly treat heart disease. Of course, the benefits of krill oil aren't limited to the cardiovascular system. In the next chapter, I will explore the ways in which krill oil helps alleviate the joint pain associated with various types of arthritis.

5

Relieving Joint Pain

When people hear the word arthritis, the image that often comes to mind is that of an elderly person's swollen and gnarled knuckles or someone bent over as they walk, always with the acknowledgement that movement for these sufferers is slow, painful, and often debilitating. The fact is that arthritis is not just a disease of old age; it strikes a broader and younger population than you might think. According to data from a recent National Health Interview Survey—an annual assessment conducted by the National Center for Health Statistics—as many as 52.5 million adults aged eighteen years or older have been diagnosed with arthritis. By the year 2030, this number is expected to increase to 67 million. The condition is higher among women than men, and of those currently diagnosed, two-thirds are under the age of sixty-five according to the Centers for Disease Control (CDC). The prevalence of arthritis increases after the very young age of thirty-five for both men and women.

Arthritis is the leading cause of disability in the United States, causing limited activity to approximately 22.7 million people who are unable to stoop, bend, kneel, or even walk. They may have difficulty grasping small objects, climbing stairs, or reaching above their head—some are unable to do these things at all. Such impairment prevents them from performing even the most basic of daily activities such as dressing, cooking, or bathing, drastically worsening their quality of life.

After presenting an overview of arthritis, this chapter will focus on the most common types along with their causes and standard treatments. While both pharmaceuticals and over-the-counter drugs are generally prescribed for arthritis, I will show you how supplemental krill oil—with its unique composition of phospholipids and omega-3 fatty acids—has been shown to improve mobility and help reduce the painful symptoms of this debilitating disease . . . naturally.

WHAT IS ARTHRITIS?

Despite the fact that arthritis impacts so many adults and children, the disease is often misunderstood. For one thing, arthritis is not a single disorder, but presents itself in more than a hundred forms and related conditions. The most common types are osteoarthritis and rheumatoid arthritis, which will be discussed in a moment. Arthritis primarily affects the joints, where one bone moves on another bone. Joints are what give us our flexibility and mobility, but they are only able to do so because of an intricate system of ligaments, cartilage, and synovial fluid.

Here's a quick and very basic lesson on how your joints work. Ligaments hold the two bones of a joint together. They are like elastic bands whose job is to keep the bones in place while the surrounding muscles help to make the joint move. Cartilage is the tough, flexible connective tissue that covers the surface of the bones to prevent them from rubbing directly against each other. (Thinking about that may remind you of chalk screeching on a chalkboard.) It is the cartilage that allows the joints to work smoothly and painlessly. In addition, the joint cavity (the space within the joint) needs hydration and lubrication, which comes in the form of *synovial fluid*. Produced by the *synovium*—a membrane that lines the joints—synovial fluid nourishes the joint and the cartilage. And that is how a healthy joint works.

Arthritis causes inflammation to the joints and the surrounding tissue. In fact, the word arthritis literally means "joint inflammation." What triggers that inflammation depends on the type of arthritis. It could be caused by cartilage that has worn away or synovial fluid that is being depleted. It may be the result of an auto-immunity (when the body's immune system mistakenly attacks itself), an infection, or a combination of many other factors, including genetic makeup, damage from a previous injury, repetitive physical motion (often from a sport), an allergic reaction, and obesity. Before further explaining how these factors can have an impact on different forms of arthritis, let's examine the two major types of arthritis: osteoarthritis, and rheumatoid arthritis.

Osteoarthritis

One of the oldest known diseases in humans, osteoarthritis (OA) is the most common form of the disease, and more likely to creep up on you as you age. Sometimes called the "wear and tear" arthritis, OA results from overusing one's joints during a lifetime. It is a progressive, degenerative disease that causes the breakdown of joint tissue. The cartilage loses its elasticity, causing it to gradually wear away in some areas and become more vulnerable to damage. In turn, the tendons and ligaments become stretched, which causes pain. The bones may eventually rub against each other, resulting in very severe pain. Typically, the disease develops gradually, starting with a bit of soreness or stiffness that most people find to be simply irritating rather than a matter of concern. Common symptoms include:

- Sore or stiff joints, particularly in the hips, knees, lower back, neck, base of the thumb, small finger joints, ankles, and big toes. Symptoms are most noticeable after inactivity (perhaps upon getting out of bed) or overuse (after physical activity).

- Stiffness after resting that disappears with movement. For instance, standing up after sitting for a long period of time or getting out of bed in the morning.

- Joint pain that is worse after activity or toward the end of the day.

For some people, osteoarthritis will never progress beyond these uncomfortable early stages. But for others, over time—and the duration of that time varies—the symptoms will become much more noticeable and debilitating.

Causes/Risk Factors

Aging joints, obesity, previous joint injury, and genetic predisposition are among the common risk factors of osteoarthritis. I've already mentioned that as a natural part of aging, we lose elasticity in our joints. Fortunately, as I will discuss later in this chapter, there are ways to maintain that mobility and decrease the risk of pain.

OBESITY

In some cases, obesity increases the risk of getting arthritis, but in all cases it makes the condition worse. One in five Americans has been diagnosed with arthritis, but according to the CDC that number jumps to more than one in three among obese people. With two out of three Americans over age twenty either overweight or obese, there is a growing concern that the percentage of people with arthritis is likely to increase significantly.

An obese person has a 60 percent greater risk of getting arthritis than those who maintain a healthy body weight. The link between obesity and arthritis is clear—the more weight placed on a joint, the more that joint will be stressed, and the more likely it will be to become worn down and damaged. This is particularly true for weight-bearing joints, particularly the knees and hips. According to research from the rheumatology division of the Mayo Clinic, every pound of excess weight exerts about four pounds of added pressure on the knees. This means that a person who is five pounds overweight is placing an extra twenty pounds of pressure on his or her knees, and the person who is fifty pounds overweight is adding an extra two hundred pounds of pressure.

PREVIOUS INJURY AND OVERUSE

Often, without even realizing it, we cause our bodies to take a beating. Whether it's from daily jogging on a hard pavement or typing on a computer for several hours at a time, we are abusing our joints. Over time, these tiny "micro-traumas" build up and can lead to arthritic joint pain.

A trauma you may have sustained when younger, like an injured knee from a car accident or a broken ankle from sliding into first base, can come back to haunt you. Years later, that injured joint is likely to be the area you start to feel pain. According to the American Academy of Orthopaedic Surgeons, damaging a joint makes your chances of developing arthritis seven times greater. As many as 15 percent of people who are diagnosed with OA have developed joint problems as a result of a past injury. There may be nothing you can do about that old football injury you got in college, but you can take natural supplements, like krill oil, to help prevent inflammation from developing and eventually leading to arthritis and joint pain.

Another issue that leads to OA is the overuse of joints, and this is particularly true for athletes. Years of straining the same set of joints with repetitive motions can lead to long-term damage. Think of the pitcher whose arm and shoulder get a constant workout, or the skier whose knees are the primary source of "abuse." Also at risk is the worker who engages in repetitive physical activities. Take the construction work, for example, whose job requires constant heavy lifting or the factory worker who runs a machine that requires a repetitive motion.

GENETICS

For some people, developing osteoarthritis is simply a matter of genetics. Although scientific researchers have not yet discovered the specific gene that causes OA, they are clear that it tends to run in families. If there's a history of osteoarthritis in your family, there is a good chance you will develop it as part of the natural aging process. On the plus side, you can take steps to prepare for it by minimizing the stress you place on your joints throughout your life. Simply having an awareness of this predisposition will also help you become better prepared to deal with OA once it develops. Later in this chapter, I will discuss how taking omega-3s in the form of krill oil can help minimize its characteristic discomforts.

Rheumatoid Arthritis

Rheumatoid arthritis (RA) is a chronic autoimmune disorder in which an overactive immune system mistakenly attacks the synovium, which lines the joints and produces lubricating synovial fluid. This leads to chronic inflammation, tenderness, pain, stiffness, and eventually the destruction of the joint. According to the Arthritis Foundation, about 1.5 million people in the United States have RA, which affects nearly three times as many women as men. In women, RA most commonly begins between ages thirty and sixty; in men, the onset often occurs later in life.

While rheumatoid arthritis can be exacerbated by a previous injury or overuse of the joints, as with osteoarthritis, it is not caused by these factors. RA is strictly an autoimmune disorder that, as previously mentioned, causes inflammation of the membranes that line the joint. The typical signs and symptoms of rheumatoid arthritis include:

- Tender, warm, swollen joints.
- Joint stiffness often followed by pain or tenderness.
- Morning stiffness that can last throughout the day.
- Numbness, tingling, and/or burning sensation in the hands.
- Fatigue.
- Low-grade fever.
- Weight loss.

Typically during the early stages of RA, the smaller joints are affected first—most commonly those at the base of the fingers and toes. As the disease progresses, symptoms often spread to the wrists, knees, ankles, elbows, hips, and shoulders. One common characteristic of RA is symmetrical joint swelling: if a joint on one side of the body is affected, the same one on the other side is affected, too. Over time, RA can cause joints to become deformed and shift out of place.

The severity of the disease varies from person to person and symptoms can change from day to day. Often sufferers experience flare-ups—periods of time lasting from a few days to a few months when the disease is more active and, therefore, more painful. Fortunately, these painful flare-ups alternate with periods of relative remission, when the swelling and pain fade or disappear. This unpredictable aspect of the disease makes it even more challenging to deal with.

Dealing with rheumatoid arthritis is a challenge made more difficult by the fact that it is caused by the body's own misguided immune system. According to studies from the National Institute of Arthritis and Musculoskeletal and Skin Diseases (NIAMS), white blood cells (agents of the immune system) target the synovium, causing inflammation. During the inflammation process, the normally thin synovium becomes thick and causes the joint to become swollen, puffy, and sometimes warm to the touch. As RA progresses, the inflamed synovium invades and destroys the cartilage and bone within the joint. This weakens the surrounding muscles, ligaments, and tendons, making them unable to do their job supporting and stabilizing the joint. Researchers at the NIAMS believe that RA begins to damage bones as early as the first year or two of the disease, which is one reason why early diagnosis and treatment are so important.

Although joint inflammation, pain, and stiffness are classic characteristics of rheumatoid arthritis, complications can occur in other parts of the body. When RA affects the wrists, the inflammation can compress the nerves that serve most of the hand and lead to carpal tunnel syndrome. Other milder symptoms by comparison can include neck pain, dry eyes, and dry mouth. The RA itself, along with certain medications for treating it, can increase the risk of osteoporosis, a condition that weakens the bones making them more prone to fracture. About 20 percent of people with RA develop rheumatoid nodules—small bumps that develop under the skin near the affected joints (often the fingers, heels, forearms, and elbows).

More alarmingly RA can compound the possibility of developing additional medical issues. In his book, *The Inflammation Revolution*, Dr. Georges M. Halpern states that while RA itself isn't fatal, sufferers are at increased risk for other diseases, like adult-onset diabetes and gastrointestinal bleeding. He continues that the "inflammation can move to the internal lining of the lungs (a condition called pleurisy) or to the peripheral nerves. Your eyes and even the lining of your heart may be affected." Many people with RA develop anemia—a decrease in red blood cell production.

Research from the NIAMS indicates that as RA develops some of the body's immune cells recognize one type of their own protein as a foreign intruder. The exact protein is unknown and may be one of any number of potential candidates. Whatever the source, cells called *lymphocytes* react to this protein, causing the release of *cytokines,* which are chemical messengers that trigger more inflammation and further destruction of the synovium. The inflammation also spreads to other areas in the body, ultimately causing not only joint damage, but also chronic pain, fatigue, and loss of function. The most significant cytokines in RA are *tumor necrosis factor* (*TNF*) and *interleukin-1,* which are both triggers of joint damage. Later in the chapter you will see how krill oil can help block these cytokines, thereby reducing inflammation and joint damage.

Causes/Risk Factors

Although the exact cause of rheumatoid arthritis is not yet known, scientists believe there is a genetic predisposition to the disease. In addition, a few possible risk factors are also helping them solve this puzzle.

GENETICS

Rheumatoid arthritis has a genetic link and can run in families. But scientists have not yet pinpointed the specific gene responsible. They have, however, discovered that certain genes called *specific human leukocyte antigens* (*HLAs*) are associated with a tendency to develop RA. They have found that people with these genes have a greater chance of developing rheumatoid arthritis than people without them. But not everyone with HLAs develops RA. Even so, researchers believe a person's genetic makeup does play an important role in determining who may develop the disease, as well as how severe it will become. Researchers at the National Institutes of Health (NIH) are constantly working on this issue.

OTHER POSSIBLE RISK FACTORS

Infectious agents like viruses and bacteria are other suspects that may trigger RA in those who are predisposed to the disease. Long-term smoking is believed to be another risk factor, as is obesity. The body's response to a stressful situation or event has also been implicated as a possible trigger.

Over 70 percent of those with RA are women. And hormonal changes or deficiencies are believed to play a role. To further support this theory, the disease often improves during pregnancy and flares up afterward. It also appears to become aggravated in women during breastfeeding and when taking oral contraceptives.

HOW ARTHRITIS IS TREATED

I wish I could say that there is a cure for arthritis, but currently, there isn't. There are, however, ways to help prevent it and delay the onset. Once the disease has manifested, a variety of treatment options are available and commonly prescribed to manage the pain. Some offer short-term relief while others are designed as long-term treatments. Although most are effective, all come with unwanted—sometimes serious—side effects. Here is a brief look at the most common treatments along with their possible risks and side effects.

Nonsteroidal Anti-Inflammatory Drugs (NSAIDs) and COX-2 Inhibitors

Prescribed to reduce joint inflammation, *nonsteroidal anti-inflammatory drugs (NSAIDs)*—like aspirin and ibuprofen—are among the most common arthritis treatments. Available in both over-the-counter and prescription strengths, NSAIDs work by blocking *prostaglandins*—hormone-like substances that contribute to the pain, inflammation, and stiffness of arthritis.

Prostaglandins are made by two different enzymes: cyclooxygenase 1 (COX-1) and cyclooxygenase 2 (COX-2). The COX-1 enzyme is normally present in a variety of tissues including areas of inflammation and the stomach. Some of the prostaglandins made by COX-1 protect the inner lining of the stomach. Prostaglandins made by the COX-2 enzyme often cause the pain and swelling of inflammation and other painful conditions. NSAIDs block both of these enzymes. Although this helps reduce inflammation, when the COX-1 enzyme is blocked, the protection of the stomach lining is lost as well.

Because some NSAIDs are low-dose and available without a prescription, many people mistakenly think they don't have any harmful side effects. Actually, some of their potential risks are quite serious, which increase with long-term use and higher dosages. Because NSAIDs block the COX-1 enzyme, which protects the stomach lining, they can cause gastrointestinal bleeding, gastritis, esophagitis (inflammation of the esophagus), and ulcers. For those with an existing kidney condition, NSAIDs may cause kidney damage or failure. They may also make heart conditions worse in those with a history of coronary artery disease.

While NSAIDs are effective in relieving the painful symptoms of arthritis, their benefits must always be considered along with their possible downsides. For the most part, I find them acceptable when used for short-term, occasional pain relief.

COX-2 inhibitors are a type of NSAID that block *only* the COX-2 enzyme. Unlike regular NSAIDs, they do not block COX-1, which protects the lining of the stomach. COX-2 inhibitors like celecoxib (Celebrex) are as effective as NSAIDs for treating inflammation and pain, but do not cause ulcers or increase the risk of stomach bleeding. In other words, they block the pain and inflammation of arthritis, but allow the COX-1 enzyme to protect the stomach lining. Even so, common side effects of COX-2 inhibitors include insomnia, abdominal pain, flatulence, headache, nausea, and diarrhea.

Acetaminophen

Acetaminophen is an analgesic drug that is commonly prescribed for arthritis pain. Unlike NSAIDs, analgesics do not fight inflammation. They reduce pain by blocking the pain signals that travel to the brain through the central nervous system. When used for an extended period, acetaminophens—like Tylenol—can have a harmful impact on the liver. Like NSAIDs, I find acetaminophens acceptable when used only occasionally and for short-term pain relief. They are not good solutions for managing pain over the long term.

Narcotics

Available by prescription only, narcotic pain relievers like codeine and oxycodone are sometimes used to manage severe arthritis pain. They do not, however, relieve joint inflammation, and can have very serious side effects—with addiction being the most significant. Developing a tolerance to the drug with repeated or long-term use is another likelihood. Other common side effects include drowsiness, constipation, nausea, and vomiting.

Corticosteroids

A class of drugs that are related to the steroid cortisone, corticosteroids are often prescribed to reduce the joint pain and inflammation associated with rheumatoid arthritis. Most often taken orally in pill form, they can also be inhaled, applied topically, given intravenously, or injected directly into the inflamed tissues. Prednisone is the corticosteroid most often prescribed to reduce the pain and inflammation associated with rheumatoid arthritis. For severe flare-ups, it can be injected into the affected joint. While both the oral and injectable forms are effective, often providing pain relief for months, both options can have side effects, particularly when taken at higher doses. Oral steroids can cause nausea, vomiting, loss of appetite, heartburn, insomnia, increased sweating, or acne. The injection can damage the cartilage in the affected area, as well as increase bruising.

DMARDs

Disease-modifying antirheumatic drugs, or DMARDs, are often used to treat people with inflammatory arthritis who have not responded to NSAIDs and who are at risk of permanent joint damage. There are several different types of these drugs, which are generally prescribed for treating rheumatoid arthritis, juvenile inflammatory arthritis, ankylosing spondylitis, psoriatic arthritis, and lupus. DMARDs work by suppressing the immune system, which is mistakenly attacking and destroying the body's joints and tissues. These drugs—which include cyclosporine (Neoral), biologics (Humira, Enbrel, Remicade), and leflunomide (Arava) among others—not only treat the symptoms, but also slow down progressive joint destruction. Side effects can include low white blood cell counts, blood or protein in the urine, nausea, and skin rashes. Treatment with these medications requires careful monitoring by a doctor.

Glucosamine and Chondroitin Sulfate

Glucosamine and chondroitin sulfate are natural substances found in and around cartilage cells. *Glucosamine* is an amino sugar that the body produces and distributes in cartilage and other connective tissue. Numerous studies have indicated that it can promote the repair of cartilage. *Chondroitin sulfate* is a complex carbohydrate produced by the body that helps cartilage retain water and elasticity, and inhibits the enzymes that break down cartilage.

In the United States, glucosamine and chondroitin sulfate are sold as dietary supplements that are regulated as foods rather than drugs. Glucosamine supplements are derived from shellfish shells, while chondroitin supplements are generally made from bovine cartilage. Clinical studies are divided about the effectiveness of either supplement. Some people report relief from arthritic pain and stiffness, but larger, well-constructed studies report no significant benefit. Glucosamine appears to be safe to consume, but studies show that when someone doesn't feel any positive effects from the dietary supplement, they tend to take more than the recommended dosage. Doing so can cause gastrointestinal problems like gas and diarrhea. More seriously, it can have a negative effect on insulin resistance, which can lead to diabetes.

Surgery

In extreme cases of arthritis in which the joints are badly damaged and treatments are not working, surgery may be a consideration. Surgery, performed by an orthopedic surgeon, may involve a number of different procedures. Removing the inflamed synovial membrane that lines the joint cavity is one common surgical process. Fusing the joint to make it more stable is another. But the most common form of surgery for arthritis is joint replacement, with hip and knee the most popular. Joint replacements are generally successful and can last an average of ten to fifteen years, often without the need for revision surgery. Downsides include the standard risks and complications inherent with any surgery; however, risks may be even greater in patients who are taking long-term steroids and other medications that affect the immune system and the ability to heal.

BENEFITS OF KRILL OIL

With the possible exception of surgery, most of the available treatment options for arthritis offer only temporary relief—which is why taking measures to prevent the progression of the disease is so important. Maintaining healthy weight is one way to avoid putting added stress on joints, especially weight-bearing joints like knees and hips. I have had patients who have seen their arthritis symptoms lessen considerably after losing as little as five or ten pounds. Exercising is another way to help build and maintain muscle and bone strength, and relieve stiffness. Basic low-impact aerobic activities like brisk walking, swimming, and biking increase cardiovascular endurance, while performing simple stretches can help improve joint flexibility and range of motion.

How else can you prevent or at least delay the development of arthritis? There is much medical evidence that the long-chain polyunsaturated omega-3 fatty acids EPA and DHA, which play a major role in reducing inflammation, can offer significant help. In fact, according to a recent study published in *Annals of the Rheumatic Diseases*, regular dietary intake of these omega-3 fats helps suppress the misguided immune system that leads to rheumatoid arthritis.

In numerous double-blind placebo-controlled studies, patients taking omega-3 supplements have shown significant decrease in the swelling, irritation, and joint pain associated with RA, as well as a reduction in the duration of morning stiffness. One major discovery by a group of researchers at Cardiff University in Wales showed omega-3s to inhibit the pro-inflammatory COX-2 enzyme.

Growing research on supplemental krill oil has shown its ability to inhibit inflammation and reduce arthritic symptoms for both osteoarthritis and rheumatoid arthritis sufferers—and within a short treatment period. One recent study published in the *Journal of the American College of Nutrition* examined the effects of krill oil (300 daily mgs) compared to a placebo on arthritis patients. After just fourteen days, inflammation markers for the krill oil group dropped 30 percent, while they rose 32 percent in the placebo group. Considering that patients taking placebo showed an increase in inflammation by 32 percent, this indicates that krill oil not only prevented inflammation, but also reduced the existing inflammation by an additional 30 percent.

In addition to exhibiting a noticeable decrease in inflammation, the patients taking krill oil showed a reduction in pain by 26 percent, stiffness by 26 percent, and functional impairment by 29 percent. These are remarkable results from a supplement. By comparison, the placebo group showed a 7 percent increase in pain, a 1 percent decrease in stiffness, and an 11 percent increase in functional impairment.

To understand krill oil's effectiveness on arthritis, it's important to first be aware of the factors implicated in inflammation. One of the most useful biomarkers (indicators) of inflammation is *C-reactive protein* (*CRP*). Increased levels of CRP in the blood indicate inflammation within the body. More specifically, in arthritic joints, CRP production indicates the release of cytokines, which, as I mentioned earlier, are chemical messengers that trigger inflammation and destruction of the synovial membrane. The most significant cytokines that trigger joint damage in RA are tumor necrosis factor (TNF) and interleukin-1. They are also found in those with osteoarthritis particularly of the knees and hips.

So how does krill oil fit into this picture? There are a number of ways it is effective. The first lies in the omega-3 fats it contains. To explain, omega-3s are transformed in the body into potent hormones called *eicosanoids,* which control a number of important functions and trigger the secretion of anti-inflammatory prostaglandins, which reduce CRP levels. This means a reduction in inflammation. Further, as you already know, the phospholipid form of the omega-3s in krill helps protect cell membranes, keeping them strong and flexible against toxic invaders. Further, krill oil naturally contains the potent antioxidant astaxanthin, which helps prevent the omega-3s from oxidizing. It is for this reason that astaxanthin is being added to a number of fish oil supplements—yet another reason that krill oil, which *naturally* contains astaxanthin, is a better choice than fish oil. Also be aware that in most cases, the astaxanthin added to fish oil is either synthetic or sourced from plants. It has been proven that krill astaxanthin is significantly more bioavailable than the type derived from plants.

While krill oil and other omega-3 supplements may not stop the progression of RA, they can significantly reduce the symptoms. In addition to protecting joints from inflammatory damage, krill oil may lower a patient's need for other treatments, including medications that have harmful side effects.

CONCLUSION

The powerful effects of long-chain omega-3 fatty acids EPA and DHA on arthritis sufferers are certainly impressive. The recent discovery of krill oil as a rich source of these beneficial fats and other important nutrients has prompted a growing number of ongoing studies. Although further research is needed to better understand how krill oil benefits arthritis sufferers, and to learn how it works in relation to other anti-inflammatory treatments, currently, there is enough evidence to support its positive effects. Already considered an impressive alternative option for treating the various forms of arthritis and other inflammatory conditions, krill's natural combination of phospholipids, EPA, DHA, and astaxanthin, may prove it to be even better than current treatments.

6

Dealing with Women's Health Conditions

So far you have learned how omega-3 fatty acids can help lower the risks of cardiovascular disease and reduce the painful symptoms of arthritis in both men and women. Researchers are also discovering that these fatty acids may be highly effective in managing a number of significant conditions that specifically affect women, including premenstrual syndrome, dysmenorrhea (painful menstruation), and menopause. Just as important, omega-3s have been found to play a vital role during pregnancy and lactation by promoting normal fetal development, preventing preterm births, enhancing infant development, and reducing postpartum depression.

This chapter will examine each of these conditions, explore ongoing research, and highlight the important health benefits that are available to women through omega-3 fatty acids.

PREMENSTRUAL SYNDROME (PMS)

Affecting women prior to their monthly menstrual cycle, premenstrual syndrome (PMS) is a hormonal disorder that is characterized by a wide range of physical and/or psychological symptoms. The American College of Obstetricians and Gynecologists estimates that at least 85 percent of menstruating women experience one or more of these symptoms, which typically occur in the days before menstruation begins and usually subside once the cycle starts.

- Abdominal bloating and pain
- Mood swings
- Fatigue
- Irritability
- Headache
- Depression
- Joint pain
- Anxiety
- Fluid retention
- Food cravings

Although some women experience fairly mild symptoms of PMS, for others, the symptoms can be more uncomfortable or even severe and require treatment. A small percentage of women—about 3 to 8 percent—experience a very severe form of PMS called premenstrual dysphoric disorder, or PMDD. Although many of the symptoms of PMDD are the same as those of PMS, for women with PMDD, the problems are so intense that they are considered disabling. Persistent, marked irritability; sudden intense mood swings; extreme sensitivity (crying); bouts of anger; significant changes in appetite (overeating or food cravings); insomnia or sleeping too much; loss of interest in usual activities; and deep depression and overwhelming feelings of hopelessness are among PMDD's most common characteristics.

Although the exact cause of PMS is not clear, fluctuating hormones—primarily estrogen and progesterone—during the menstrual cycle are primary suspects. Estrogen begins to rise slowly after a woman's period ends, peaks around two weeks later, and then begins to drop again when menstruation begins. Progesterone levels remain low during the first half of the cycle, increase a bit after ovulation, and then drop at the end of the cycle. These hormonal shifts are likely contributors to the mood swings and physical discomforts associated with PMS.

When estrogen levels decline, there is a change in the body's *neurotransmitters*—chemical messengers in the brain that communicate information throughout the body. Some neurotransmitters, like norepinephrine and dopamine, are considered *excitatory* and responsible for stimulating the brain, while others, like serotonin, are considered *inhibitory* and help create calmness and balance. (See "Understanding Neurotransmitters" on page 103.) When estrogen decreases, so do the levels of serotonin and dopamine. A promotor of "happy feelings" and a sense of well-being, serotonin helps regulate mood, appetite, and sleep. It also involves cognitive functions, including memory and learning. Dopamine is involved with attention span and focus, as well as motivation. Low levels of both serotonin and dopamine have been cited as the reason for many mild to moderate cases of depression. Decreased estrogen levels may also cause an increase of the neurotransmitter norepinephrine, resulting in stress, anxiety, and irritability.

When determining the causes of PMS, it's easy to understand why hormonal imbalance is such an important consideration. There are, however, other possible contributors, including low blood-sugar levels, caffeine consumption, and oral contraceptives (due to the synthetic progesterone they contain). Deficiencies in certain vitamins and minerals, like vitamin B_6, calcium, and magnesium, can worsen PMS symptoms. Eating salty foods, which can cause fluid retention, and drinking alcohol, which can cause mood disturbances, can also make the discomforts of PMS worse.

Common Treatments

There are a number of ways to treat PMS, from dietary adjustments and lifestyle changes to natural alternatives and medications. I am always in favor of making lifestyle adjustments and trying natural approaches before turning to pharmaceuticals.

Exercise

Regular exercise can help reduce and manage PMS symptoms. Thirty minutes of daily physical activity like brisk walking, jogging, bicycling, or swimming can improve symptoms like fatigue and depressed mood. Exercise prompts the release of endorphins—the "feel-good" brain chemicals—which help lift moods and boost energy.

Dietary Adjustments

Several dietary modifications can help decrease PMS symptoms. Eating smaller meals more frequently throughout the day can reduce bloating and fullness. Limiting the intake of salty foods is another way to reduce bloating. Avoiding coffee and other caffeinated drinks, which can increase anxiety and insomnia, is recommended, as is consuming alcohol, which can act as a depressant. To avoid blood-sugar fluctuations, stay away from anything processed, including foods or beverages made with refined ingredients like white sugar, white flour, and white rice.

Stress Reduction

Getting enough sleep is one important way to reduce stress and help alleviate some of the symptoms of PMS. Muscle relaxation exercises, deep breathing techniques, yoga, and massage are all effective stress-reducing methods. You can also help fight stress by simply doing the things you enjoy, such as reading a book, watching a movie, or pursuing a hobby.

Medications

Several medications may be prescribed to relieve PMS symptoms, depending on their severity. To lessen the physical discomforts of breast tenderness and cramping, non-steroidal anti-inflammatory drugs (NSAIDs), like aspirin and ibuprofen, are commonly prescribed. Although NSAIDs can offer relief, they can also cause potentially serious side effects, like gastrointestinal bleeding, which increase with overuse or long-term use.

For women with severe PMS or PMDD, which can be debilitating, doctors may recommend antidepressants. Most antidepressants work by changing the levels of neurotransmitters in the brain. The ones most commonly prescribed are *selective serotonin reuptake inhibitors (SSRIs)*, which affect the neurotransmitter serotonin. They work by blocking the reabsorption of serotonin into the brain, thereby making the chemical more available to the body. SSRIs include the brands Prozac, Zoloft, Paxil, Lexapro, and Celaxa.

Of course, as with all pharmaceuticals, these antidepressants are not without side effects, which may include the following: nausea, dizziness, nervousness and anxiety, insomnia, weight gain or loss, vomiting, dry mouth, diarrhea, and reduced sexual desire. More seriously, some antidepressants can cause dangerous reactions when combined with certain medications or even herbal remedies. When certain pain relievers (aspirin, ibuprofen, naproxen, warfarin) are combined with SSRIs, there is an increased risk of abnormal bleeding. And most serious, in some cases, children, teens, and young adults may experience an increase in suicidal thoughts or behavior when taking antidepressants. The FDA has instructed all drug manufacturers to add this "black box warning" to the labeling of all antidepressant drugs. (For information about other classes of antidepressants, see page 101.)

Benefits of Omega-3s and Krill Oil

Research shows that omega-3 fatty acids in general—and krill oil, in particular—provide an effective natural treatment for relieving a number of symptoms commonly associated with PMS, including bloating, headache, breast tenderness, loss of concentration, and depression.

As reported in the *Alternative Medicine Review*, Canadian researchers conducted a double-blind study designed both to evaluate the effectiveness of krill in the management of PMS and to compare the effectiveness of krill oil with that of fish oil. The subjects included seventy women who were diagnosed with PMS and experienced symptoms that included anxiety, lack of concentration, nervousness, bloating, headache, breast tenderness, and feeling of sadness and mild depression. One group received omega-3 fish oil, and the other, krill oil. The groups were assessed after forty-five days and after ninety days, and at both times, it was found that krill oil was significantly more effective than fish oil in the management of breast tenderness, joint pain, and the emotional symptoms of PMS. The subjects who took krill also used significantly fewer painkillers and reported an increase in alertness, energy, and general well-being.

Krill oil's superior results were attributed to the phospholipid form of the omega-3s in krill oil, which allows them to be better absorbed than those in fish oil's triglyceride form. The final results of the study suggest that krill oil can significantly reduce the physical and emotional symptoms of premenstrual symptoms and are more effective in the management of PMS than fish oil.

Researchers don't fully understand how omega-3 fatty acids reduce the physical symptoms of PMS, but at least some of the effects are believed to be caused by the anti-inflammatory properties of the fatty acids. Following ovulation, omega-6 fatty acids are released in the body, triggering inflammation. This, in turn, increases the incidence of breast tenderness, joint pain, and other common symptoms of PMS. The consumption of supplemental omega-3 fatty acids triggers the release of anti-inflammatory substances, which create an environment that reduces inflammation-related problems.

The emotional problems experienced during the premenstrual period are usually attributed to fluctuating hormone levels and their impact on those neurotransmitters that affect mood. Since omega-3 fatty acids appear to regulate hormones and neurotransmitters by correcting the balance of fatty acids in the body, fish and marine oils may reduce PMS's emotional symptoms by influencing hormone and neurotransmitter levels. In addition, as you will learn in Chapter 7, when the body has a rich supply of omega-3 fatty acids, mental well-being is significantly improved in several different ways. Researchers in the Depression Clinical and Research Program (DCRP) at Massachusetts General Hospital found that EPA and DHA—the long-chain omega-3s found in krill oil—are as effective as antidepressants in improving mood, and various studies have supported the researchers' conclusion that omega-3s can fight depression and help people deal better with daily stresses. (For more information about omega-3 fatty acids and depression, see page 107.) It makes sense, then, that omega-3s can help improve mood and emotional stability in the weeks prior to menstruation.

DYSMENORRHEA

Dysmenorrhea is the medical term for the painful menstrual cramps that many women experience in the lower abdomen right before menstruation begins—as prostaglandins peak, causing uterine contractions—and for two or three days after it starts. This is the most commonly reported menstrual disorder. More than half of women who menstruate suffer from this pain for one or two days each month, and for some women, the cramps they experience can be disabling.

The medications most commonly prescribed for menstrual pain are NSAIDS, which reduce the amount of prostaglandins and lessen their effects. Some women, however—including those with bleeding disorders, asthma, liver damage, stomach disorders, and ulcers—should not take NSAIDS.

Fortunately, research has shown that omega-3s can help lessen the painful cramps that accompany menstruation. In Denmark, a survey among Danish women indicated that a diet high in fish oils lessened menstrual cramping. A double-blind placebo-controlled study was then designed to test this hypothesis. Seventy-eight women who suffered pain during menstruation were given omega-3 supplements or a placebo, and after three months, the women receiving omega-3s reported significant improvements in pain. As you learned on page 89, a study conducted in Canada also showed that omega-3s reduce pain related to menstruation. The Canadian study also indicated that krill oil provides a level of pain reduction superior to fish oil, enabling participants to use fewer painkillers.

PREGNANCY AND FETAL DEVELOPMENT

Research published in *Reviews in Obstetrics & Gynecology* emphasizes that adequate consumption of omega-3 fatty acids is essential during pregnancy and in the months after birth, and that the most biologically active forms of omega-3s are DHA and EPA derived from marine sources. These fatty acids have benefits for not only the developing child but also the mother.

Promoting Normal Fetal Development

Omega-3 fatty acids, especially DHA, are critical for the fetal development of the brain, eyes, and central nervous system, especially during the third trimester, when fetal brain cells are being created at an extraordinary rate (more than 250,000 nerve cells per minute). Depending on the mother's consumption of omega-3s prior to and during pregnancy, these fatty acids are passed to the baby via the placenta. If the pregnant woman does not have adequate supplies of DHA in her body, her fetus' brain will have trouble keeping up with the growing demand for DHA building blocks. (For more about the infant's need for DHA to prevent childhood neurological problems, see page 112 in Chapter 8.)

Data derived from both observational studies and double-blind placebo-controlled studies indicate that adequate omega-3 consumption during pregnancy, through either high-seafood diets or nutritional supplements, results in improved neurological development in the child. Investigators used a variety of tests—measures of a child's developmental milestones, language development, problem solving, and more—to compare the outcomes among infants whose mothers were supplemented with fish oil or had high-seafood diets to the outcomes among infants whose mothers consumed lower amounts of omega-3s. The results showed that babies whose mothers received higher levels of omega-3s scored higher on developmental tests. Indeed, these fatty acids were found to be so important to the normal development of the brain and eyes that researchers suggested that a mother's omega-3 requirements may increase above normal during pregnancy.

Although seafood seems to provide the developing infant with the same benefits offered by omega-3 supplements, seafood can also contain organic mercury and other harmful toxins. For this reason, the FDA counsels pregnant women to limit seafood consumption to two small portions per week. Therefore, to avoid toxicity, omega-3 supplements are a better means of ensuring optimal infant development.

Preventing Preterm Births

Preterm birth—the birth of an infant before thirty-seven weeks of pregnancy—is the leading cause of infant death. It is also the chief cause of long-term neurological problems in children.

The idea that omega-3 supplementation may prevent preterm birth originated from studies of the Faroe Islands. The population of the Faroe Islands has a higher intake of marine foods than the population of nearby Denmark, and babies born on the islands have a higher birth weight at term than babies born in Denmark as well as thirty-three other countries. As the result of this observation, trials were designed to compare the pregnancies of women who received fish oil capsules, DHA supplementation, or DHA-enriched eggs with women who received no omega-3 supplementation. A number of studies showed that women with higher omega-3 fatty acid consumption had longer gestational length and a reduced risk of preterm births. At this time, researchers do not feel that the study results have been conclusive, but it is believed that daily omega-3 supplementation taken to optimize fetal brain development may have the additional advantage of increasing gestational length.

Enhancing Infant Development During Lactation

Research shows that after the birth of her child, a nursing woman's consumption of omega-3s—especially DHA—continues to provide her baby with nutrients needed not only for neurological development but also for protection against certain common infant disorders. In one study, when lactating women received 200 mg of DHA per day over a period of four months, their breast-fed infants performed better on the Bayley Psychomotor Development Index than did the infants of women who received a vegetable oil supplement. In another study, women who had allergies or had a spouse or child with allergies were given either omega-3 fatty acids or a placebo, beginning in pregnancy and continuing for three or four months into lactation. The infants of the omega-3-

supplemented mothers showed a significantly decreased risk of developing both food allergies and IgE-associated eczema.

So far, studies have given us only a taste of the benefits provided to infants by omega-3 fatty acids. As research into the effects of omega-3s continues, we may learn more ways in which these beneficial nutrients can ensure infant health.

Reducing Postpartum Depression

Approximately 10 to 20 percent of childbearing women suffer from perinatal or postpartum depression. More than the "baby blues," this is a clinical depression that can strike pregnant women, women who have just given birth, and women who have given birth over the last year. While antidepressants can help, many women who are pregnant or lactating are understandably reluctant to take medications that may affect their infants.

As you will learn in Chapter 7, a rich supply of omega-3 fatty acids appears to significantly improve mental health. Because a developing fetus requires a good supply of these nutrients and draws them from the mother, pregnancy decreases a mother's stores of these fatty acids. While observational studies have suggested an association between low concentrations of omega-3s and a greater risk for postpartum depression, so far, controlled studies have failed to show a clear benefit of omega-3 supplementation to the prevention of depressive symptoms after childbirth. Further research is needed to determine if omega-3 fatty acids can make a significant contribution to the emotional well-being of new mothers.

MENOPAUSE

Menopause is the time in a woman's life that begins twelve months after her last menstrual period. Caused by lower levels of reproductive hormones, especially estrogen, it usually occurs in a woman's forties or fifties. In the United States, the average age for menopause is fifty-one.

Although menopause is a natural event, low levels of estrogen can result in many uncomfortable and disruptive symptoms, including hot flashes, mood swings, depression, insomnia, vaginal dryness, urinary tract infections, thinning and decreased elasticity of the skin, and the loss of sex drive. About 10 to 15 percent of menopausal women seek medical help. At one time, hormone therapy was routinely used to treat menopausal symptoms, but after a large clinical trial indicated that this treatment posed serious health risks, including higher risks of cancer and cardiovascular disease, its use became less common. Antidepressants are also sometimes effective in reducing symptoms, although these drugs are also associated with side effects.

Fortunately, omega-3 fatty acids appear to offer some relief without dangerous risks and unwanted side effects. In 2005, two small but well-controlled Italian studies set out to determine if omega-3s can help relieve hot flashes. The researchers attributed a "progressive and highly significant reduction" in hot flashes to the fatty acid supplements, possibly through their influence on nerve cell membranes or neurotransmitter function. A few years later, a Canadian study was published in *The American Journal of Clinical Nutrition*. At Université Laval, 120 menopausal women ages forty to fifty-five were divided into two groups. One group was given an EPA supplement of marine origin, and the other was given sunflower oil supplements without EPA. Both before and after the eight-week test period had ended, the omega-3 group experienced significant relief of psychological stress and mild depression. The women who were suffering from hot flashes also enjoyed improvement. Researchers observed that the reduction of hot flashes was equivalent to that obtained with phytoestrogens and antidepressants.

While more studies need to be performed, it appears that supplementation with omega-3 fatty acids can offer significant relief to women struggling with the symptoms of menopause.

CONCLUSION

Even when the symptoms of PMS and menopause are mild, they can disrupt a woman's life, and when these symptoms become severe, they can be truly debilitating. It's good to know that omega-3 fatty acids—a natural product—can help reduce premenstrual and menopausal problems without causing disturbing and dangerous side effects.

Perhaps most exciting, omega-3s have been proved vital during pregnancy and lactation, when a bountiful supply of DHA and EPA helps ensure normal infant development. While a number of studies have shown success using seafood-rich diets and fish oil supplements, krill offers a source of omega-3s that is pure, potent, and easily absorbed and used by the body. Future studies are sure to reveal more of the important benefits that omega-3s and krill oil can provide for women.

7

Alleviating Depression

Depression is a psychological condition characterized by feelings of sadness, disinterest in daily life, feelings of guilt or low self-worth, disturbed sleep or appetite, low energy, and poor concentration. This mental health problem can become chronic or recurrent, and severe cases of depression can lead to a withdrawal from friends and family, feelings of futility, irrational outbursts of anger, and even suicide. Chronic depression can also trigger a wide variety of physical symptoms, including gastrointestinal problems, back pain, chest pain, joint pain, and headaches. Any existing pain or physical condition may be worsened by depression.

Depression is one of the most common mental disorders not only in the United States, but throughout the world. Recently, it was estimated that 17 million U.S. adults age eighteen or older have at least one major depressive episode each year, and that 350 million people globally suffer from some form of depression. And this disorder takes a heavy toll. According to the World Health Organization, depression is among the leading causes of disability, affecting about 121 million worldwide.

After presenting an overview of depression, this chapter will discuss possible causes and standard treatments. Pharmaceuticals, psychotherapy (talk therapy), and lifestyle changes have long been used to manage depression, but studies now show that supplemental krill oil can be an effective natural therapy for this all-too-common problem.

WHAT IS DEPRESSION?

Most people have felt sad or depressed at various times. Depression can be a normal reaction to the loss of a loved one, the end of a relationship, or another distressing life situation. But when this feeling includes a sense of hopelessness and continues for weeks, it may be the condition known as *clinical depression, major depression*, or *major depressive disorder*.

A mental health provider is best able to determine whether clinical depression is present. The *Diagnostic and Statistical Manual of Mental Disorders (DSM)*, published by the American Psychiatric Association, states that for the diagnosis of clinical depression, five or more of the following symptoms must be experienced over a two-week period, nearly every day, for most of the day:

- A depressed mood, such as feeling sad or tearful.

- Greatly lessened interest or lack of pleasure in all or most normally pleasurable activities.

- Significant unintentional weight loss or weight gain, or a marked decrease or increase in appetite.

- An inability to sleep or an increased desire to sleep.

- Restlessness or slowed behavior that is noticeable to other people.

- Fatigue or a great loss of energy.

- Feelings of inappropriate and excessive guilt or worthlessness.

- Difficulty in making decisions, thinking, or maintaining focus.

- Repeated thoughts of death or suicide.

The above symptoms of depression must be so severe that they cause obvious problems in day-to-day activities such as work or school, and they interfere with relationships. In addition, they cannot be caused by the direct influence of a substance such as a medication or alcohol.

Causes and Risk Factors

Depression is a complex disease that can occur for a number of reasons. The following factors may increase the risk of experiencing depression:

- Past physical, sexual or emotional abuse.

- Certain medications, such as the antiviral drug interferon alpha and corticosteroids.

- Grief over loss of a loved one.

- An inherited tendency toward depression.

- Major life events and changes such as graduating from college, getting married, moving, starting a new job, getting a divorce, losing a job, or retirement.

- A serious illness such as cancer.

- Abuse of substances such as alcohol.

- Nutritional deficiencies.

Sometimes, the cause of depression seems obvious. This is especially true after someone experiences the loss of a loved one or undergoes a traumatic event. But in other cases—such as a nutritional deficiency or use of a medication—it can be more difficult to determine the origin of this condition. Many experts believe that depression is most likely caused by a combination of factors. For instance, a depressive episode can be triggered by a genetic predisposition acting together with an upsetting event such as the loss of a job.

Before we turn to the topic of treatment, it should be noted that another common cause of depression is premenstrual syndrome (PMS), which many women experience during their menstruating years. However, this chapter focuses on clinical depression, which lasts more than two weeks, while PMS-related depression generally occurs during the two weeks prior to menstruation and is relieved when menstrual flow begins. To learn about PMS, see Chapter 6.

HOW DEPRESSION IS TREATED

Although many people who suffer from depression never seek treatment, even when the illness is severe, the vast majority can benefit from some type of therapy. It's important to understand, though, that there is no definitive way to cure depression, and that what works for one person might not work for another. Often, different treatments or a combination of approaches must be tried before significant improvement is experienced.

The most common treatments for clinical depression are psychotherapy and medication. Lifestyle changes and supplements can also offer relief.

Psychotherapy

Psychotherapy, also known as *talk therapy,* is usually the first form of treatment recommended to treat depression. Most people think of therapy as individual counseling in the form of one-on-one sessions, conducted by a professional therapist who might be a psychiatrist, psychologist, licensed clinical social worker, or nurse practitioner. Since the patient's close relatives are usually affected as well, there is also the option of family counseling, which treats the entire family. A third alternative is group counseling, which gives patients an opportunity to meet other people who are also struggling with depression.

After the initial evaluation, the therapist usually chooses one of two approaches: cognitive therapy or psychodynamic therapy. *Cognitive therapy* is based on the idea that during depressive episodes, the affected individual has dark thoughts that can take over and distort views of reality, contributing to the depression. In this form of therapy, the therapist helps the patient learn new ways to react to situations and offers problem-solving techniques. Over time, this can change the way the individual sees the world.

Psychodynamic therapy is based on the assumption that individuals become depressed because of unresolved conflicts that exist on an unconscious level and often stem from childhood. By encouraging the depressed patient to talk about these experiences, the therapist helps the individual understand the causes of the conflict and guides him or her in coping better with them.

Talk therapy can be a powerful treatment for depression by identifying internal conflicts and providing stress relief, coping skills, and a new perspective on life. But it is effective only when the patient is willing to do the hard work necessary to change his or her behavior and outlook. Even if the individual is very motivated, psychotherapy may not be enough to resolve severe depression, and medications may be prescribed to provide relief.

Medications

As discussed in the treatment section for PMS (see page 88), antidepressants are commonly prescribed for depression. These medications are administered by a psychiatrist, general practitioner, or nurse practitioner, and are considered safest when accompanied by some form of psychotherapy. Drug therapy may be short-term or long-term, depending on the severity of the condition.

It has been estimated that one in ten Americans take antidepressants. But it often takes both time and patience to find the drug that works best for the individual, and in some cases, these drugs can cause troubling side effects.

Many different medications can be used, alone or in combination, to treat depression. The most widely prescribed antidepressants include selective serotonin reuptake inhibitors (SSRIs), serotonin and norepinephrine reuptake inhibitors (SNRIs), tricyclic antidepressants (TCAs), and monoamine oxidase inhibitors (MAOIs).

The most commonly prescribed antidepressants are the *selective serotonin reuptake inhibitors (SSRIs)*. These drugs ease depression by affecting the *neurotransmitters*—the chemicals used by the brain to communicate with other brains cells as well as cells throughout the body. (To learn more about neurotransmitters, see the inset "Understanding Neurotransmitters" on page 103.) By preventing reabsorption (reuptake) by the brain of the neuro- transmitter serotonin, SSRIs make more of this chemical available in the brain, which, in turn, boosts mood. As you'll learn in the discussion below, all antidepressants work by changing levels of one or more neurotransmitters.

Some of the best-known SSRIs now in use are Prozac, Zoloft, Paxil, Celexa, Lexopro, and Pexeva. These medications share sim- ilar side effects, which can include, but are not limited to, nausea, nervousness, dizziness, drowsiness, insomnia, weight gain or loss, vomiting, diarrhea, and reduced sexual desire or sexual dysfunc- tion. Like all antidepressants, they must be taken under the super- vision of a physician.

Another class of frequently prescribed antidepressants is *the serotonin and norepinephrine reuptake inhibitors (SNRIs)*. Similar to the SSRIs just discussed, these drugs elevate mood by blocking absorption of the neurotransmitters serotonin and norepineph- rine, and also block the reuptake of other brain chemicals. Com- monly used SNRIs include Cymbalta, Effexor XR, and Pristiq. Among the possible side effects of SNRIs are nausea, dry mouth, dizziness, excessive sweating, fatigue, anxiety, difficulty urinat- ing, constipation, loss of appetite, and sexual problems.

Tricyclic antidepressants (TCAs), sometimes call *cyclic antide- pressants*, are among the earliest antidepressants developed. Although they have generally been replaced by antidepressants that cause fewer side effects, they are still prescribed and can be effective. Like the class of medications discussed above, they work by blocking the absorption of the neurotransmitters serotonin and norepinephrine. Some of the TCAs now in use are Amitriptyline, Amoxapine, Norpramin, Doxepin, Tofranil, Pamelor, Vivactil, and Surmontil. Possible side effects of cyclic antidepressants include dry mouth, blurred vision, constipation, drowsiness, increased appetite leading to weight gain, lightheadedness resulting from drops in blood pressure, disorientation or confusion, tremor, irreg- ular heartbeat, and sexual dysfunction.

Understanding Neurotransmitters

Throughout the discussion of antidepressants, you read how these drugs were designed to relieve depression by changing the levels of neurotransmitters that are available to the brain. But what exactly are neurotransmitters, and what do they do in the body?

Neurotransmitters are chemicals that relay signals between nerve cells, or *neurons,* to transmit information throughout the brain and body. The brain uses these chemicals to regulate not only mood, but also heartbeat, sleep, and a range of other vital activities. When the correct amounts of these chemicals are present, your brain is in sync with your body. But when the levels of these chemicals are either too high or too low, problems can occur.

Dozens of neurotransmitters have been identified, all of which can have a number of effects and can work in combination with one another and with other substances in the body. This discussion introduces some of the best-known, most important brain chemicals.

There are two major types of neurotransmitters: excitatory and inhibitory. *Excitatory neurotransmitters* promote the transmission of information from one neuron to another and have a stimulating effect on the body. Some of the major excitatory neurotransmitters include dopamine, epinephrine, and norepinephrine. *Dopamine*—which is special because it's also an inhibitory neurotransmitter—plays a critical role in the control of the brain over the body's movements, maintains focus and motivation, regulates the flow of information within the brain, and stabilizes brain activity. It also provides feelings of enjoyment, thereby motivating you to repeat certain behaviors. When the level of dopamine is too high or too low, you may experience problems such as depression, lack of focus, or impaired memory. *Epinephrine* and *norepinephrine,* also called *adrenaline* and *noradrenaline,* are related hormones that have similar functions. They both constrict arteries, open airways in the lungs, increase the rate and force of heart contractions, and perform other activities. High levels of these chemicals can cause anxiety and irritability, while low levels can cause depression, fatigue, and other problems.

Inhibitory neurotransmitters decrease the brain's ability to transmit messages and have a calming effect on the body. Some of the major inhibitory neurotransmitters are serotonin, GABA (gamma-aminobutyric acid), and dopamine. *Serotonin* controls hunger cravings, regulates the sleep cycle, manages pain, calms anxiety, stabilizes mood to help maintain positive feelings, and promotes cognitive functions such as memory and learning. Low levels of this neurotransmitter can cause food cravings, insomnia, depression, fatigue, and loss of concentration. *GABA,* which is sometimes referred to as "nature's Valium," calms the brain, prevents anxiety, and lowers blood pressure. Deficiencies of GABA can lead to anxiety, insomnia, and hypertension. You've already read about *dopamine,* as it is both an excitatory and an inhibitory neurotransmitter. It stabilizes brain activity, provides feelings of enjoyment, helps maintain focus and attention span, and regulates both physical movement and the flow of information in the brain. Insufficient dopamine can result in problems ranging from depression to cravings for junk food. Levels of inhibitory neurotransmitters can be depleted by the use of stimulatory substances, like caffeine, and by the excessive firing of excitatory neurotransmitters in the brain.

Because neurotransmitters are involved in all body functions and play a vital role in emotional well-being, a number of symptoms, some of which are quite serious, can result if these chemicals are not present in the body at the right levels. Unfortunately, it is estimated that nearly 90 percent of Americans have less-than-optimal levels of these chemicals as the result of chronic stress, poor diet, prescription and recreational drug use, environmental toxins, and other factors.

Monoamine oxidase inhibitors (MAOIs) were the first antide-pressants to be developed, and like tricyclic antidepressants, they have generally been replaced by newer medications that involve fewer side effects. They work by removing the neurotransmitters serotonin, dopamine, and norepinephrine from the brain, which makes more of these chemicals available. Unfortunately, they also affect other neurotransmitters, especially those affecting diges-tion. Currently, the MOAIs in use include Marplan, Nardil, Emsam, and Parnate. Typically, these drugs require dietary restric-tions because when paired with certain foods, MOAIs can cause dangerously high blood pressure. Other possible side effects include dry mouth, nausea, diarrhea, constipation, drowsiness, insomnia or other sleep disturbances, dizziness or lightheaded-ness, weight gain, sexual dysfunction, involuntary muscle jerks, and difficulty starting the flow of urine.

Antidepressants may help relieve some of the symptoms of moderate and severe depression. But depression can be compli-cated, and while there can be chemical imbalances within the body that can lead to the illness, often, there are also underlying problems like emotional trauma. Furthermore, as you've just learned, antidepressants come with side effects and safety con-cerns. This is why other treatments should be considered.

Lifestyle Changes

Lifestyle changes can help ease depression or at least keep symp-toms at bay. These changes by themselves probably can't beat depression, but by enhancing the health of your mind and body, they can effectively complement other treatments and help pre-vent future depressive episodes.

Exercise increases your body's natural production of feel-good chemicals like the neurotransmitter serotonin and the hor-mone endorphin. Research shows that exercising for thirty minutes or more a day can help alleviate depression, boost mood, reduce stress, and lead to more restful sleep.

Adequate sleep is essential to good mental and physical health. Sleep deprivation has been show to exacerbate irritability, moodiness, sadness, and fatigue. Unfortunately, common complications of depression include the inability to fall asleep and the tendency to wake in the middle of the night and then remain awake. Sometimes, a calming bedtime routine, used consistently at the same time every evening, can help the body relax, improving both the quality and quantity of sleep.

Eating well-balanced meals throughout the day helps maintain energy and minimize the mood swings caused by a high-sugar diet. For mental well-being, nutritionists suggest that your diet incorporate the complex carbohydrates found in fresh produce and the beneficial fatty acids found in certain fish.

Good stress management, which combats anxiety and depression through calming experiences and thoughts, should be part of everyone's life. Each day, build in time to watch a movie, read a book, listen to music, write in a journal, or pursue a hobby. Also keep in regular contact with friends and family as a means of avoiding isolation and enriching your world.

Nutritional Supplements

For people who want to avoid the side effects of antidepressants or who simply wish to add a natural weapon to their anti-depression arsenal, supplements are a good option. Certain herbs and vitamins have been shown to offer some relief from symptoms of depression. For example, some of the B complex vitamins—specifically, B_6 and B_3—have been found to improve mood by affecting levels of the neurotransmitter serotonin. Theanine, an amino acid derivative found in green tea, has long been known to trigger the release of the calming neurotransmitter GABA. Calcium, iron, selenium, and zinc have also been linked to mood improvement.

The herb St. John's wort has been shown to have a positive effect on various neurotransmitters, including serotonin and dopamine/norepinephrine, in the treatment of mild to moderate depression. A Cochrane database review of twenty-nine studies involving 5,489 patients with mild to moderate depression found St. John's wort to be superior to placebo and similarly effective as some antidepressants but with fewer side effects.

When it comes to natural supplements, perhaps most promising are the omega-3 fatty acids, which have been shown to support emotional well-being. (Read more about this below.)

If you do decide to try supplements, first check with your doctor or therapist. Even natural remedies can have side effects and serious drug interactions. And always be sure your doctor is aware of any supplements you are taking when a new medication is prescribed or prior to any surgery.

BENEFITS OF OMEGA-3s AND KRILL OIL

If you or a loved one suffers with depression, you know that it can be difficult to get this disorder under control, and that it is not unusual for depression to recur over time. Psychotherapy can be helpful, but relief can be slow in coming, and antidepressants, although often effective, can cause a host of side effects, some of which are serious. Fortunately, there is a great deal of evidence to support the use of omega-3 fatty acids to prevent and treat mood disorders, including depression.

The link between mental health and omega-3 fatty acids is hardly surprising, as the human brain is 60-percent fat and rich in omega-3s, particularly in the membranes of certain brain cells. About 8 percent of the brain is comprised of these fatty acids. Large epidemiological studies have repeatedly shown that when reduced levels of omega-3s are found in red blood cells and serum, brain function is affected and depression occurs. In a recent analysis, researchers from the National Institutes of Health (NIH) found that low blood levels of the omega-3s raise suicide risk as much as 62 percent. On the other hand, a rich supply of omega-3s appears to significantly improve mental well-being. In a Norwegian study of nearly 22,000 participants, it was found that those who regularly took cod liver oil, which is high in omega-3s, were roughly 30-percent less likely to suffer symptoms of depression than those who didn't use this oil—and that those individuals who had been taking the oil longest were the least likely to suffer from mood disorders. Omega-3s have also been found to help people who have already been diagnosed with depression. In a recent study at the Royal College of Surgeons in Ireland, omega-3 fatty acids were randomly given to patients who had repeatedly harmed themselves. At the end of the three-month study period, those patients who received fatty acids supplement showed a significantly improved ability to deal with daily stresses and a reduced incidence of depression.

A good deal of research has specifically cited eicosapentaenoic acid (EPA) and docosahexaenoic acid (DHA)—the two long-chain omega-3 fatty acids—as making a real difference in people suffering from depression. A research director in the Depression Clinical and Research Program (DCRP) at Massachusetts General Hospital stated that EPA and DHA are considered to be as active as antidepressants in improving mood. Studies have supported that supplements which include both of these acids—which occur together in nature in various ratios—seem most effective at helping people with depression.

EPA and DHA are thought to help improve mood in a variety of ways. EPA, for example, is believed to enhance mood by reducing inflammatory processes in the brain. DHA appears to have far-reaching hormonal effects by increasing the amount of corticotropin-releasing hormone (CRH), which has moderating effects on the emotions. Both EPA and DHA seem to aid in the transmission of messages between brain cells, possibly by boosting the levels of certain neurotransmitters. A recent study also showed that older people who consume more omega-3s have an increased amount of gray matter, and that most of the newer tissue development is found in the section of the brain that is specifically associated with feelings of happiness. Although researchers do not yet understand the precise mechanisms involved, ample studies have demonstrated that omega-3s have a significant effect on mental health, and especially on mood.

Rich in both EPA and DHA, krill oil is the best source of omega-3s when seeking to prevent or treat depression and other mood disorders. As you learned in Chapter 3, the bioavailability of dietary omega-3 fatty acids improves when they are bound to phospholipids. This means that the EPA and DHA provided by krill oil are more effectively absorbed first through the intestinal wall, and then by the tissues that need them—including the tissues of the brain. The phospholipids in krill contain another nutrient, choline, in the form of phosphatidyl-choline, which is essential to brain development and health. Moreover, krill oil provides the antioxidant astaxanthin, which not only prevents the DHA and EPA fatty acids from oxidizing but also passes on free radical-fighting benefits to the brain tissues, helping avoid inflammation and other damage.

While krill oil may not, on its own, be able to prevent or treat depression in all cases, its combination of omega-3 fatty acids, phospholipids, and astaxanthin has shown a powerful ability to help maintain brain health and substantially improve mood.

CONCLUSION

In even its mildest forms, depression can have a profound impact on your life, and when severe, this condition can be truly debilitating. Because it can have far-reaching effects, you should always consult a physician if you suspect that either you or a loved one is experiencing this disorder. However, ample studies have demonstrated that EPA and DHA, the omega-3 fatty acids abundant in krill oil, can help maintain and restore emotional health. While research on the impact of omega-3s on brain health and mood disorders is relatively new, the results to date have been more than promising, making krill oil a worthy weapon in the war against depression.

8

Additional Health Benefits

The last few chapters have focused on the omega-3 fatty acids in supplemental marine oils, highlighting krill oil and its superior advantage in helping to both prevent and treat heart disease, arthritis, PMS and other menstrual problems, and depression. Not surprising, krill oil can also provide benefits in many other areas of your health. In fact, an understanding of this miraculous nutrient will change the way you view—and treat—many of our nation's most common conditions and diseases.

This chapter explores krill oil's potential to help relieve some of the most widespread health epidemics that face Americans today, including neurological-based diseases like attention deficit disorder and Alzheimer's; inflammatory conditions like lupus and irritable bowel syndrome; cancer; and skin and eye problems. Krill oil can even have a positive impact on overall aging. While this amazing nutritional supplement may not be able to alleviate all your health problems, it can certainly be a valuable addition to your daily regimen, particularly if you suffer from any of the conditions discussed in the following pages.

NEUROLOGICAL-BASED DISORDERS

The brain is 60-percent fat, with 8 percent of this organ composed of omega-3 fatty acids. The most abundant of the brain's fatty acids is docosahexaenoic acid (DHA), which plays an important role in brain development, in the transmission of messages from one brain cell to another, and in the protection of the brain from oxidative stress. It is therefore not surprising that reduced levels of omega-3s, and especially DHA, are associated with structural problems and impaired thinking, and that supplementation with omega-3s shows tremendous promise in the prevention and treatment of attention deficit hyperactivity disorder, dementia, and Alzheimer's disease.

DHA is not the only reason krill oil has such a positive impact on neurological conditions. As you already know, krill oil, unlike fish oil, contains the high-potency antioxidant astaxanthin. Astaxanthin has the unique characteristic of being able to cross the blood-brain barrier—a kind of barricade that prevents foreign "harmful" substances in the blood from entering the brain. Because astaxanthin is able to cross this barrier, its antioxidant activity can help prevent the brain and central nervous system from the damage caused by free radicals.

Attention Deficit Hyperactivity Disorder (ADHD)

Researchers have found that DHA is essential for the developing brain, both during gestation and afterwards. Omega-3s accumulate in the brain during fetal development, and babies born to mothers who have higher blood levels of DHA show advanced attention spans through their first and second years. On the other hand, studies conducted by Purdue University suggest that children who are deficient in omega-3 fatty acids are much more likely to display behavior problems such as *attention deficit hyperactivity disorder (ADHD)*, a common childhood disorder marked by hyperactivity, difficulty in maintaining focus, and trouble in controlling behavior. ADHD affects 3 to 10 percent of school-aged children, and an estimated 60 percent of them will continue to have disruptive symptoms into adulthood. The most common class of drugs used to treat ADHD are stimulants like Ritalin, but many of these pharmaceuticals have the potential to cause disturbing side effects such as depression, dizziness, and insomnia.

Fortunately, researchers have found that supplementing with omega-3s—at any age—can make a positive difference in attention span and cognitive powers. Members of the International Organization of ADHD conducted a study in which subjects who took 500 mg of krill oil every day for six months showed a 60-percent increase in concentration, a 39-percent improvement in the ability to focus, and almost a 50-percent increase in social skills. In another trial, thirty patients between the ages of ten and thirty-two, all of whom were known to have had ADHD for at least three years, were administered 500 mg of krill oil daily. The subjects' Barkley executive function scores—which measure the individual's ability to exercise self-control, perform goal-directed behavior, and solve problems—were noted both before and after the three-year trial. After completing the treatment, patients showed a significant improvement in all areas.

Another research study published by Neptune Technologies & Bioressouces showed that thirty adult ADHD patients who used 500 mg of krill oil daily for six months reported a 60-percent increase in the patients' concentration and a 47.8-percent increase in planning skills.

These study results offer hope to both adults and children with ADHD as well as other problems with concentration and attention span. The indication is that krill oil can improve focus and a range of cognitive abilities when taken consistently over a period of time. Potentially, this can help reduce the need for those drugs now prescribed (particularly to young children) for treating attention deficit disorders. Of course, further research is required to better understand the dosage and the long-term effects of omega-3s on both children and adults.

Alzheimer's and Dementia

Just as omega-3s are important to brain development in infants and children, they are known to be vital to brain health and cognitive powers in the middle-aged and elderly.

For many years, it was assumed that brain shrinkage, the death of nerve cells, and impaired cognitive powers, which are all characteristics of dementia, are unavoidable, progressive, and irreversible for many people. Statistics seem to bear this out, as one in three seniors is affected by some form of dementia—a group of symptoms that affects memory, thinking, and social abilities—with Alzheimer's disease being the most common cause of this disorder. Although medications such as Aricept are used to temporarily improve symptoms and even slow the progression of the basic disease process, there is currently no cure for this widespread and debilitating disorder.

Research, however, shows that dementia may not be inevitable. Studies focusing on omega-3s indicate that nutrient deficiencies may account for many age-related problems of the brain. In a Framingham Offspring Study of middle-aged subjects,

Aging and Omega-3 Fatty Acids

Throughout this book, you have learned how omega-3 fatty acids can help you avoid or relieve certain disorders that are associated with getting older, such as cardiovascular disease and Alzheimer's disease. The fascinating truth is that in addition to combating many of the problems of aging, these beneficial fats may actually slow the aging process.

As you get older, your DNA—your genetic material—becomes increasingly damaged, especially at the *telomere,* which is the repeating sequence of DNA found at the end of the chromosome. Sometimes compared to "plastic tips of shoelaces," the telomere helps protect the genes so that they can divide properly. Nevertheless, over time, as cells divide and replicate, the telomeres lose some of their length. Eventually, the telomeres become so short and damaged that cells can no longer divide, resulting in poor cell health, disease, and eventual cell death.

Researchers continue to debate the factors that may contribute to the rate at which telomeres become shorter. It has been suggested that in addition to age, other factors, such as infection, smoking, lack of exercise, and obesity may all damage telomeres.

lower levels of DHA and EPA were associated with lower brain volume, accelerated structural aging of the brain, and reduced cognitive ability. On the other hand, the majority of studies published to date indicate that increased fish consumption resulting in higher levels of DHA and EPA can lower the risk of dementia and cognitive decline. One study found that older people who consumed more omega-3 fatty acids actually had increased brain volume. Another clinical trial found that daily supplementation with DHA in older adults caused an improvement in learning and memory function over the twenty-four-week study period.

Researchers have offered several theories to explain the link between the increased consumption of omega-3s and improved brain health. Both DHA and EPA have been found to have

What *is* known is that many age-related conditions—including heart disease, excessive weight gain, diabetes, and cartilage loss—are linked to telomere shortening. This is because as telomeres age, they create a trio of problems, including inflammation, oxidative stress, and the aging of immune cells, all of which spur the development of disease and the rate at which the entire organism ages.

Amazingly, a study has shown that a high consumption of omega-3 fatty acids can slow the rate at which telomeres shorten. Published in the *Journal of the American Medical Association,* the study was conducted at the University of California in San Francisco. Over a period of five years, researchers followed the progress of 608 subjects with coronary heart disease, evaluating them via blood tests to determine their levels of the omega-3 fatty acids DHA and EPA. At the end of the study period, it was found that those who had the highest levels of omega-3 fatty acids had the slowest rate of telomere shortening.

The exact mechanism that slows damage to the telomeres is not known, but evidence suggests that people with a high consumption of omega-3s actually age more slowly than people with lower levels of the fatty acids, and therefore have the potential to live longer, healthier lives.

favorable effects on the body's vascular system, including reduced blood pressure, reduced inflammation, lower serum triglyceride levels, and lowered risk of thrombosis (blood clots within blood vessels). Since these vascular disorders are associated with a higher risk of dementia, omega-3s may delay brain aging and cognitive problems such as memory loss. Omega-3s may also help protect the brain by reducing oxidative damage, combating the inflammation characteristic of Alzheimer's disease, and protecting the ability of the brain to transmit messages across the synapses.

Studies are ongoing regarding the relationship between omega-3 fatty acids and brain health, but so far, research has shown that omega-3s may have a unique capacity to combat Alzheimer's and age-related dementia. Because krill oil is rich in DHA, EPA, and the antioxidant astaxanthin, and because it is more easily absorbed by the tissues of the brain than are fish oils, it offers great promise as a means of preserving both brain volume and brain function.

CHRONIC INFLAMMATION

Chapter 1 discussed the effectiveness of omega-3 fatty acids in reducing chronic inflammation and the broad spectrum of disorders it can cause or exacerbate. In Chapters 4 and 5, you learned in greater detail how omega-3s—especially in the form of krill oil—can make a positive difference in the treatment of two of these health problems, cardiovascular disease and joint pain. Below, you'll discover how krill oil can positively affect other chronic inflammation-related conditions, as well.

Before you learn about the amazing effects that krill can have on inflammation, it's important to understand a phenomenon that you may notice as you read the following pages. Most of the inflammatory diseases discussed—including lupus, Crohn's disease, and psoriasis—are also autoimmune disorders, meaning that the immune system is mistaking its own tissues as foreign and launching an attack on the body. This is not a coincidence. There are more than eighty types of autoimmune diseases, and the classic sign of these disorders is inflammation, which can cause redness, heat, pain, and swelling. In other words, inflammation and autoimmune disease are closely associated.

Lupus

Lupus is a chronic autoimmune disease in which the immune system attacks the body's organs and tissues, leading to painful or swollen joints, fever, skin rashes, kidney or heart problems, and extreme fatigue. The Lupus Foundation of America estimates that at least 1.5 million Americans have lupus, with more than 16,000 new cases reported annually across the country. At least 5 million people throughout the world have a form of the disease.

Lupus strikes mostly women of childbearing age—ages fifteen to forty-four. However, men, children, and teenagers develop lupus, too. The cause of lupus is not known, and there is no cure for the disease. Steroids and other drugs are often prescribed to manage the condition, but these medications can have serious side effects.

Fortunately, omega-3 fatty acids appear to offer a measure of relief. In one study involving fifty-two patients with active lupus, subjects were given either fish oil supplements, a copper supplement, a copper supplement plus fish oil, or a placebo. At the end of the six-month study period, copper appeared to offer no benefits, but all of the patients who had received fish oil supplements experienced improvements in inflammation, fatigue, and overall quality of life. Some of the subjects who were taking fish oil along with their usual steroid treatments were actually able to reduce their steroid dosage. The researchers concluded that individuals with lupus could benefit either from taking omega-3 supplements or from increasing their consumption of fatty fish.

Asthma

Asthma is an inflammatory condition in which the airways narrow, swell, and produce extra mucus, causing chest tightness, shortness of breath, wheezing, and coughing. A major public health problem, it affects an estimated 25 million Americans and about 300 million people worldwide, and the numbers are increasing every year. For some individuals, it is a nuisance. For others, it can be life-threatening.

Because asthma is such a widespread and often serious problem, a large number of medications have been developed in an effort to control it. These medications include, but are not limited to, inhaled corticosteroids (steroids) such as Asmanex; oral leukotriene modifiers such as Singulair; inhaled long-acting beta agonists such as Serevent; and fast-acting rescue inhalers such as Maxair. Some of these medications have a relatively low risk of side effects, but others can cause serious reactions at the time of use or create long-term problems after repeated use. For instance, long-term reliance on steroids can lead to depression, mood swings, osteoporosis, hypertension, high blood sugar, glaucoma, and an increased risk of cataracts.

Fortunately, omega-3s offer new hope for asthma sufferers. In a study at Indiana University, researchers found that adults with mild to moderate persistent asthma who took omega-3 supplements daily for three weeks enjoyed 64-percent improved post-exercise lung function, enabling a 31-percent decrease in the use of emergency inhalers. While this study specifically examined exercise-induced asthma, in which individuals experience inflammation of the airways (bronchoconstriction) immediately after exercise, researchers believe that the anti-inflammatory effects of the omega-3s could also benefit people with other types of asthma.

Cancer

Cancer poses a major health problem in the United States and throughout the world. According to the American Cancer Society, over 1.5 million new cases are diagnosed each year in the U.S., and although recent years have shown a decline in deaths, over 500,000 people in the United States die annually from this insidious disease. Worldwide, over 14 million adults are diagnosed with cancer each year, with 8 million annual deaths.

Chronic inflammation has been found to be a causative factor in many types of cancer. In general, the longer that inflammation continues, the higher the risk of the disease. It seems reasonable, therefore, that the use of anti-inflammatory omega-3 fatty acids may help prevent the development of cancer. In fact, in a study reported in the *International Journal of Cancer*, women without breast cancer were found to have higher breast tissue levels of omega-3s than women with the disease.

Research also indicates that omega-3s can help fight cancer once it begins. In a study published in *Carcinogenesis*, researchers at Queen Mary, University of London tested the effects of omega-3s on *in vitro* samples of squamous-cell carcinoma (SCC), which causes the majority of skin cancers. It was found that the fatty acids—and especially EPA—block the growth of the cancer and induce cell death in both early and late-stage forms. Just as important, the omega-3s do not appear to affect normal cells.

Further research, presented at the 2014 ISSFAL Biennial Congress, is especially interesting because it compared krill oil's ability to fight cancer with fish oil's ability to fight cancer. In the study, conducted at Victoria University in Melbourne, Australia, laboratory plates of human colorectal cancer cells were treated with different solutions, including commercial krill oil, fish oil, and olive oil, and were examined after twenty-four, forty-eight, and seventy-two hours. Of the three solutions, krill oil was found to be the most effective at inhibiting the proliferation of the cancer cells (meaning that it reduced or delayed the growth and spread of the cancer), showing significant anti-cancer effects after twenty-four, forty-eight, and seventy-two hours. Although the fish oil matched the EPA and DHA concentrations in the krill oil, it did not inhibit proliferation at all three time-points.

Clearly, the study of the use of omega-3 fatty acids to combat cancer is in its infancy. It is hoped that future research will indicate which forms of cancer respond to omega-3s and how these fatty acids in krill oil can best be used in the war against cancer.

Inflammatory Bowel Disease (IBD)

More than 1.5 million Americans suffer from inflammatory bowel disease (IBD), which involves the chronic inflammation of all or part of the digestive tract. IBD primarily includes *ulcerative colitis,* which is characterized by inflammation of the lining of the colon (large intestine) with ulcer formation; and *Crohn's disease,* which is most commonly characterized by inflammation at the end of the small bowel (ileum) and the beginning of the colon. Both of these disorders can cause cramping and abdominal pain, bloody diarrhea, and weight loss. Both can also be debilitating, and for some people, they can lead to life-threatening complications, including colon cancer.

The goal of treatment for IBD is to reduce the inflammation that triggers symptoms. A number of drugs are used, with the most common being corticosteroids, which block the effect of the chemicals that kick-start inflammation, and immune system suppressors, which suppress the immune response that causes inflammation. When drug therapy is not effective, surgery may be necessary. It is estimated that over half of the people who suffer with Crohn's require at least one surgery, and surgery may also be used to treat ulcerative colitis.

A number of studies have shown that fish oil supplements can have positive effects in the treatment of IBD. In one uncontrolled study, six patients with ulcerative colitis were given EPA supplements for twelve weeks. A significant improvement of symptoms was noted. In the first large placebo-controlled study of IBD, ninety-six ulcerative colitis patients were given either EPA or an olive oil placebo, along with conventional treatments. The EPA treatment group had improved symptoms and a reduced use of steroids. Similar studies of patients with Crohn's disease have shown that omega-3s can reduce both symptoms and the number of relapses.

Although krill oil was not used in the human studies described above, animal research supports the use of krill oil as a weapon against IBD. The *Scandinavian Journal of Gastroenterology* detailed a study in which rats fed a diet supplemented with krill oil were significantly protected from markers of experiment-induced colitis. Researchers concluded that krill oil provides the digestive system with both anti-inflammatory and antioxidant effects.

Psoriasis and Other Skin Problems

Omega-3 fatty acids have long been known to offer multiple benefits for the skin. They are responsible for the health of the skin cell membrane, which allows the passage of nutrients into the skin, permits the movement of wastes out of the skin, and makes skin appear more youthful and wrinkle-free by enabling the cells to hold water. Omega-3s provide additional benefits by reducing the body's production of inflammatory compounds, which play a part in the development of nearly every skin condition from acne to vasculitis. And if you've wisely replaced fish oils with krill oil, your skin will have another advantage, since krill oil contains the powerful antioxidant astaxanthin. By neutralizing the free radicals caused by ultraviolet (UV) rays, environmental pollutants, and chemical toxins, astaxanthin can help protect your skin from the damage that can lead to aging, inflammation, and even skin cancer.

Because of the many skin-related benefits of omega-3s, researchers believe that these fats will prove useful in the prevention and treatment of a range of skin disorders. Already, studies have shown that omega-3 fatty acids can make a positive difference in the treatment of psoriasis.

A chronic inflammatory skin condition, psoriasis is the most prevalent autoimmune disease in the United States, affecting as many as 7.5 million people. It is estimated that 125 million people throughout the world suffer from psoriasis.

Plaque psoriasis, which is the most common form of this disorder, is marked by red patches of skin covered with silvery scales; dry cracked skin that may bleed; and itching, burning, or soreness. Like most autoimmune disorders, psoriasis involves flare-ups alternating with periods of remission. Currently, there is no cure for psoriasis, although several treatment options are available, including topical creams, light therapy, and oral medications.

A study published in the *Journal of Clinical, Cosmetic, and Investigational Dermatology* in 2011 showed that omega-3 fatty acids can make a significant contribution to the treatment of psoriasis. Researchers evaluated the effectiveness of omega-3s as a nutritional supplement in patients with mild to moderate plaque psoriasis. Of the thirty patients in the study, fifteen were given a topical psoriasis treatment only, while the remaining patients were given both the topical drug and an omega-3 fatty acid supplement. While both groups showed improvement, the group that took the omega-3s showed the greatest improvement, with fewer lesions, less scaling, and less area affected by the disorder.

DRY EYE SYNDROME AND OTHER EYE PROBLEMS

Dry eye syndrome (DES) is characterized by a chronic lack of sufficient lubrication and moisture on the surface of the eye as well as inflammation of the ocular surface. A common problem worldwide, its effects can include reduced vision; difficulty in reading; difficulty in driving at night; and persistent feelings of dryness, scratchiness, and burning. Topical solutions designed as artificial tears are the most widely used therapy for dry eyes, but these products provide relief that is temporary and incomplete at best. Other products designed to restore the tear film, such as Restasis, offer more lasting improvement for some individuals, but fail to alleviate symptoms for others. For that reason, DES has been the subject of a great deal of research in the last few years.

Because omega-3 fatty acids have anti-inflammatory properties and provide nutrients essential to eye health, a double-blind, placebo-controlled study was designed to examine the role of omega-3 fatty acids in dry eye syndrome. Published in the *International Journal of Ophthalmology,* the study divided 518 patients with dry eye syndrome into two groups. One group received a placebo while the other group received EPA and DHA supplements. Four patient visits were arranged over a three-month period to evaluate each subject through visual acuity tests; routine tear function tests; subjective reports of symptoms, including feelings of itching, burning, a gritty sensation, and blurring; physical examinations of the eyes; and other means. At the end of the study period, it was found that omega-3 supplementation had modified the inflammatory process and altered the secretions of the meibomian glands in the eyelids, improving the "staying power" of

tears. The improvement was most marked in patients with meibomian gland disease and chronic blepharitis (inflamed itchy eyelids). The researchers concluded that supplementation with
omega-3 fatty acids offers important benefits to individuals suffering from dry eye syndrome and related disorders.

Studies are ongoing to explore the part that omega-3s may
play in protecting the eyes from macular degeneration, the leading cause of vision loss among people age fifty and older. While
higher blood levels of EPA and DHA due to diets rich in fatty fish
are associated with a lower risk of neovascular ("wet") age-related macular degeneration, so far, nutritional supplementation with
omega-3s has not been shown to prevent or slow progression of
the disease.

What is more important is that krill oil contains astaxanthin,
which has been proven to be more than 550 times more powerful
than vitamin E for neutralizing free radicals. Astaxanthin crosses
the blood-brain barrier and the blood-retinal barrier. This means
it is able to provide antioxidant and anti-inflammatory protection
for the eyes, brain, and central nervous system, reducing the risk
for cataracts, macular degeneration, blindness, dementia, and
Alzheimer's disease. Studies combining krill oil with lutein, an
important eye nutrient, are currently underway. Researches
hypothesize that krill oil's high content of phospholipids and
antioxidants will help increase the bioavailability of the lutein.

CONCLUSION

The healing powers of omega-3 fatty acids are truly remarkable
and far reaching. Earlier chapters have detailed the use of this
vital nutrient in the prevention and treatment of such disorders as
cardiovascular disease, joint disease, premenstrual syndrome, and
depression. This chapter has presented some of the lesser-known
ways in which omega-3s can improve your well-being. As you've
learned, omega-3 fatty acids offer real hope in the battles against
neurological problems like ADHD and Alzheimer's disease;
chronic inflammatory and autoimmune disorders such as lupus
and Crohn's disease; common eye and skin diseases; and even

some forms of cancer. Perhaps most encouraging is that high levels of DHA and EPA have been associated with a slower progression of the aging process, which means that omega-3s may be able to prevent a wide spectrum of age-related disorders. While fish oil supplements have shown positive effects in a great many studies, there is good reason to believe that krill oil, which can be more easily absorbed and used by the body, would have more significant effects. Moreover, krill oil offers astaxanthin, a powerful antioxidant not found in fish oils.

Now that you know about the wide-ranging benefits of krill, the time has come to put the information you have read into practice. Chapter 9 will help you determine if you have a deficiency in omega-3s, guide you in making dietary adjustments that will boost your consumption of omega-3-rich foods, and—most important—show you how to use krill oil supplements not just to safely and effectively relieve current health disorders, but also to lower the risk of future problems.

9

Krill Oil Guidelines

At this point, you know the importance of omega-3s for good health, and recognize krill oil as a superior source of these valuable nutrients. This chapter is designed to present some helpful guidelines for making supplemental krill oil part of your daily regimen. Starting off, the chapter provides you with information on assessing your current omega-3 status, followed by some of the ways you can increase that status through diet and supplements. The chapter concludes with a presentation of recommended krill oil dosages and considerations, along with helpful buying and storing tips.

DETERMINING YOUR OMEGA-3 STATUS

As you already know, chronic inflammation is the underlying cause of most medical problems—you could say it's the number-one enemy of good health. With omega-3 fatty acids playing a significant role in reducing inflammation, maintaining adequate levels is very important. We now know that there are a number of signs and symptoms to help you make this determination. Start by paying attention to your body. Recognizing the symptoms that may indicate an omega-3 deficiency is key. Among the most common symptoms include the following:

- Dry skin
- Cracked nails
- Dry, lifeless hair
- Fatigue
- Depression

- Dry eyes
- Lack of motivation
- Aching joints
- Difficulty losing weight
- Forgetfulness

If you have tried to lose weight by going on a low-fat or fat-free diet, and you have also eliminated fish and seafood from your diet, you are at an increased risk of being deficient in omega-3s.

Another important step is maintaining a proper ratio of omega-3s and omega-6 fatty acids. In Chapter 1, you learned that omega-6 fats—found in meats and animal products like eggs, as well as nuts, seeds, and vegetable oils like soybean, corn, peanut, grape seed, safflower, and sunflower—are essential for good health when consumed in small amounts. But too much can cause inflammation. To reduce this risk, it's important to consume omega-6 fats with an equal (or close to equal) amount of omega-3s. For general good health, that ratio should be between 3:1 and 6:1. Unfortunately, for the average American, who tends to eat significantly more omega-6s than needed, this ratio is closer to 20:1—an unhealthy balance that has led to the growing incidents of chronic inflammatory diseases and conditions. It's important to decrease the intake of omega-6s, while increasing the intake of omega-3s.

Discovering if you have the right balance of omega fats can be done with a simple blood test, which can usually be performed through a local lab with a doctor's prescription. My test preference is the Boston Heart Lab Fatty Acid Balance Test, which is done after fasting for at least eight hours. This test, which you can have prescribed by your doctor, provides a comprehensive evaluation of all important fatty acid levels. Home test kits, which involve mailing a blood sample (from a finger prick) to a lab, are also available. Results are then mailed to you. If you are considering this option, be aware that in some states it is illegal to send blood samples through the mail.

This type of blood test measures the presence of omega-6 and omega-3 fats in your red blood cells. The results represent a fairly accurate reflection of their ratio throughout your body, including your brain. If the ratio of omega-6 to omega-3 is higher than ten, your body is in a state of inflammation. The ideal ratio is below three.

If the test results indicate that an adjustment is necessary, together with your doctor, you can formulate an effective diet/supplement plan.

MAKING DIETARY AND SUPPLEMENTAL ADJUSTMENTS

Maintaining a wholesome balance of omega-6 and omega-3 fats is largely about making the right food choices. Basically, it's a matter of minimizing your consumption of omega-6 foods and increasing your intake of omega-3s.

Ideally, although omega-6 fats are essential in small amounts, remember that too much can lead to chronic inflammation and a number of often-serious health problems. Minimize your intake of the following foods, which are sources of omega-6 fats:

- Safflower oil, grape seed oil, sunflower oil, corn oil, and soybean oil.

- Nuts and seeds, particularly pine nuts, walnuts, Brazil nuts, and pecans.

- Snacks foods like potato chips, popcorn, cheese puffs, etc., made with omega-6 oils.

- Highly processed foods like pastries, cookies, and other baked goods.

- Red meat

- Dairy products like butter

Just as important as minimizing your intake of omega-6 foods is maintaining an adequate intake of omega-3s, particularly those containing eicosapentaenoic acid (EPA) and docosahexaenoic acid (DHA)—the two long-chain fats that are the most easily utilized by the body. As you saw in Chapter 2, although there are many omega-3 food sources, fatty cold-water fish are among the best sources of desirable EPA and DHA. The American Heart Association recommends eating this type of fish at least two times a week. The best choices include:

- Anchovies
- Herring
- Mackerel
- Wild salmon

- Sardines
- Trout
- Fresh tuna

Unfortunately, if you are like most Americans, you don't eat the recommended amount of fish that is necessary to obtain the EPA and DHA fatty acids for optimal health. For this reason, taking a dietary omega-3 supplement is a good way to help ensure that you are getting enough. Fish oil supplements have long been among the most popular omega-3 sources. They are not, however, without their downsides. Part of a billion-dollar industry, fish oil supplements vary greatly, ranging in quality from pharmaceutical- to inferior-grade products.

Some supplements have been found to contain significantly fewer omega-3s than what is stated on the label. Recently, a company called LabDoor analyzed thirty of the top-selling fish oil supplements for levels of omega-3 fatty acids. It found that six of those products contained 30 percent less than what was stated on their labels. Further, the products contained measurable amounts of mercury, with three recording 50 percent or greater of the allowable mercury content per serving.

Another serious problem with fish oil is that it oxidizes easily, which causes it to spoil. The way fish oil supplements are produced makes a difference. Those that are manufactured under nitrogen (meaning they are not exposed to oxygen) stay fresh longer. Those that are exposed to oxygen during the manufacturing process become spoiled. Although the amount of spoilage (and even contamination in some cases) depends on the raw materials themselves along with the processes of extraction, refining, concentration, encapsulation, storage, and transportation. In the LabDoor study, a number of the tested oils did not pass the freshness test.

Researchers at New Zealand's Crop and Food Research Institute also tested fish oil brands from countries all over the world. They discovered that a significant number of tested capsules had begun to oxidize. According to the researchers, when fish oil becomes oxidized, it loses its potency, which minimizes its benefits. But even more critical, rancid fish oil is associated with serious health conditions including hardening of the arteries and increased blood clotting—the very conditions that the omega-3 supplement is supposed to help prevent.

It is in your best interest to use caution when taking fish oil supplements. Consumers are urged to check with the USP Dietary Supplement Verification Program, a nonprofit group that does regular spot checks on supplements and provides a seal to the ones that meet its requirements. Products that carry the seal are considered good quality. The problem is that the program is voluntary, and many supplement manufacturers do not participate in it.

While fish oil has been the most common supplemental source of omega-3s, the recent discovery of krill oil as another rich source of EPA and DHA—with even greater benefits than fish oil—offers consumers another option.

THE ULTIMATE OMEGA-3 SUPPLEMENT

Although I have talked about the benefits of krill oil in other chapters, I want to summarize a few important points about this powerful supplement, including how it differs from fish oil.

There are a number of ways in which krill oil differs from (and is superior to) fish oil as a source of omega-3s. Perhaps most significant is that the majority of long-chain EPA and DHA fats contained in krill oil are attached to phospholipids—a form that makes them more absorbable than the triglyceride form, which is the structure found in most fish oils. This phospholipid structure allows for an easier entrance of the omega-3s into cells and facilitates a more efficient transfer to target tissues such as the brain, heart, liver, and kidneys.

The phospholipids in krill oil have the added bonus of containing another vital nutrient, choline in the form of phosphatidyl-choline (PC). To further explain, the omega-3s in fish oil's triglyceride form are not able to be used by the body immediately. First, they must be attached to a molecule of phosphatidyl-choline by the liver. Only then is the body able to absorb them. Unlike fish oil, krill oil already contains the biologically active form of PC, so it can be absorbed by the body immediately as is. This better delivery and absorption of DHA and EPA make them significantly more bioavailable than those in fish oil.

In addition to phosphatidyl-choline and a rich abundance of readily available EPA and DHA in phospholipid form, krill oil contains vitamin E, vitamin A, and the potent antioxidant astax-anthin. Clinically shown to protect cells against the harmful effects of oxidation, astaxanthin helps preserve the stability of krill oil, protecting it against the effects of free radicals. When exposed to oxygen, fish oil spoils easily. Krill oil, on the other hand, is significantly protected against spoilage thanks to valuable astaxan-thin. And when compared to fish oil, the antioxidant potency of krill oil was found to be significantly greater.

Another benefit of krill oil over fish oil is that it is more easily digestible. About 80 to 85 percent of fish oil is never absorbed in the intestine, which causes about half of those who take it to experience reflux, burping, and an unpleasant fishy aftertaste. Conversely, the quick absorption of krill oil eliminates or minimizes these unpleasant side effects.

Recommended Serving Guidelines

Krill oil is considered a dietary supplement. The FDA has not established recommended daily allowances for omega-3s (like those found in supplemental krill oil and fish oil). The standard daily suggested krill oil dosage—based on clinical studies on joint, heart, women's health, and cognitive health—are as follows:

General health: 500 to 1,000 mg (1 g)

Joint health: 300 mg

Heart health: 1,000 mg for patients with coronary heart disease

Premenstrual/menstrual relief: 1,000 mg

Cognitive health: 500 mg

Take krill oil as directed on the label or as prescribed by your doctor. Do not exceed the recommended amounts.

BUYING GUIDELINES

Krill oil is readily available in drugstores, supermarkets, natural foods stores, and vitamin shops. It is also available through practitioners and can be purchased online. Knowing what to look for before purchasing this supplement will help ensure that you are choosing a quality product. It's important to check labels. You want to choose a product that is pure krill oil—one that does not contain preservatives, flavorings, sugars, or other fillers. Capsule size, cost, and even the packaging are other factors to consider.

Size Matters

Supplemental krill oil generally comes in 300 mg, 500 mg, and 1,000 mg (1 g) soft capsules. Size is a consideration when determining the value of the product based on the price you're paying for it.

According to Wellwise.org—whose mission is "to provide unbiased, accurate, and authoritative information regarding healthy living and nutrition"—deciding product value for price requires a bit of math. Simply divide the price of the product by the total milligrams it contains. The cost may be less for a bottle of 300 mg capsules that contains a total of 27,000 mg; however, since most manufacturers recommend a daily krill oil dose of 1,000 mg, you would need to take three capsules (which would still be 10 percent less than the suggested amount). Smaller capsules at a lower price are not necessarily your best value.

What's Inside?

When shopping for supplemental krill oil, be sure to read labels. Look for the following ingredients: omega-3s, preferably with a breakdown of EPA and DHA; astaxanthin; and phospholipids. And take note of their amounts. (See the table on page 133.)

Phospholipids are krill oil's most important ingredient. As you've learned, the valuable omega-3s in krill oil are attached to phospholipids (unlike the triglycerides found in fish oil). In this phospholipid form, they are more easily absorbed by the body, which is one of the qualities that makes krill oil so beneficial. Without phospholipids, krill oil would be nothing more than ordinary fish oil.

Phospholipids should make up approximately 40 percent of the total dose. This means that a 1,000-mg dose of krill oil should contain around 400 mg of phospholipids. If phospholipids do not appear on the label (or if they are not contained in this minimum amount), the quality of the product is questionable. In other words, instead of pure krill oil, the product is likely a mixture of other ingredients, usually fish oil.

Be sure to note the amount of omega-3s stated on product labels. And keep in mind that although omega-3s may be listed, if phospholipids are not also listed, you will have to ask yourself where the omega-3s came from. Chances are they were derived from fish oil, which means they are less effective. Fish oil is also less expensive, so if the cost of the krill oil is much less than other brands and phospholipids do not appear on the ingredient list, the product is likely to be inferior.

Finally, check for astaxanthin—the potent antioxidant that is naturally present in krill. Many products do not list astaxanthin on their labels because the product contains too little of it. A good-quality krill oil supplement should contain at least 0.75 mg (750 mcg) of this beneficial ingredient per 1,000-mg dose. And before purchasing, don't forget to check the "use by" date on the package. This will help guarantee product freshness and effectiveness.

The following table presents the ingredients to look for in pure krill oil, along with their recommended minimum amounts.

These totals are based upon a 1,000-milligram (mg) serving, which is the suggested daily recommendation by most manufacturers for general good health. Keep in mind that these amounts are approximate and considered minimums. Also note that daily values for these ingredients have not been established by the FDA.

RECOMMENDED MINIMUM INGREDIENT AMOUNTS	
INGREDIENT	RECOMMENDED MINIMUM AMOUNT*
Phospholipids	400 mg
Omega-3 Fatty Acids	250 mg
Eicosapentaenoic acid (EPA)	135 mg
Docosahexaenoic acid (DHA)	75 mg
Astaxanthin	0.75 mg (750 mcg)

*Amounts are based on a 1,000-milligram (mg) serving.

A Word About Price

One obvious difference between krill oil and fish oil is the cost, with krill oil being more expensive. One of the primary reasons for this difference in price is that krill, which come primarily from southern Antarctic waters, cost more to catch and process than fish. For a 1,000-mg dose of pure Antarctic krill oil, you can expect to pay anywhere from 60 to 99 cents. It's important to keep this in mind, because if you come across a brand that is significantly cheaper, there is a good chance that it is not a pure product. Many good-quality brands will state on labels that the product is, in fact, 100 percent krill oil.

STORAGE GUIDELINES

Krill oil is best stored at room temperature in a dry place. When exposed to temperatures higher than 100°C (212°F) or lower than 50°C (34°F), its therapeutic properties lose their effectiveness. Also make sure the bottle is air-tight. Exposure to humidity can lead to capsule leakage, causing them to stick to each other.

Krill Oil Supplementation and Safety Issues

Suppliers of krill oil (as well as fish oil) must produce a Certificate of Analysis—an authenticated document issued by an accredited firm or individual certifying that the product has been tested for quality and purity.

Microbial tests are done to ensure that the product does not contain salmonella, *E. coli,* or staphylococcus, according to the standards set by the US Food and Drug Administration (FDA). For the presence of heavy metals, like mercury, lead, and arsenic, standards have been set by the World Health Organization (WHO) and the Environmental Protection Agency (EPA) regarding the allowable parts per million (ppm) that can be contained in any substance that is to be ingested. This has been particularly important in light of the growing awareness of these contaminants in seafood. Because these contaminants are found throughout the environment, they accumulate in the food chain. Krill's place at the very bottom of the food chain—coupled with the fact that they live in the deep pristine South Ocean waters—minimizes their accumulation of these toxins.

Krill's clean environment also minimizes the presence of harmful dioxins like polychlorinated biphynels (PCBs). The FDA has set the acceptable PCB level in fish at 2 ppm. With reported findings of PCBs in krill at very low parts per *trillion* (ppt), the levels are nearly undetectable and easily fall within the FDA safety standards.

Tests for rancidity are also performed in compliance with standards established by the Global Organization for EPA and DHA Omega-3 (GOED).

As with any supplement, when purchasing krill oil, be sure to look for brands by reputable manufacturers that have been carefully tested. This will ensure selection of high-quality products that offer the best possible results.

CAUTIONS AND CONTRAINDICATIONS

There have been no reports of serious adverse side effects from taking krill oil. A number of manufacturers have certified their products as Generally Regarded As Safe (GRAS) by the FDA. Occasional bouts of mild digestive distress, including indigestion and loose stools, have been reported in studies. There are, however, certain precautions that must be taken for certain health conditions and possible drug interactions.

Like fish oil, krill oil has possible blood-thinning effects. For this reason, it is not advised for anyone taking a prescription anticoagulant (blood thinner) like warfarin (Coumadin) or a pain reliever like aspirin chronically without first consulting with a doctor. In fact, people who are at risk of bleeding complications for any reason should consult a physician before taking fish oil or krill oil.

Although omega-3s are believed to offer significant health benefits to pregnant women, as well as the fetuses they are carrying (see Chapter 6), it is always best to first consult with a physician. This advice is also recommended for those with a severe liver condition.

Finally, because krill is a marine creature, anyone with an allergy to shellfish should proceed with caution. While there have been many cases in which taking krill oil did not elicit an allergic response, it is still best to steer clear until you have discussed this with your doctor.

CONCLUSION

Now that we've come to the end of this chapter (and of this book) you know the importance of omega-3s for good health. In this chapter, you've learned how to recognize the signs of a possible omega-3 deficiency, as well as ways to improve it—which can be as simple as making a few dietary adjustments and including supplemental omega-3s as part of your daily regimen.

You have also seen how krill oil is a superior source of these (and other) valuable nutrients. This chapter has presented helpful guidelines for taking this supplement, along with purchasing tips, including cost and what to look for on labels.

For decades, medical researchers have extolled the many health benefits of these omega-3 fatty acids, and now you have come to know them, too. While fish oil has long been viewed as the best supplement for obtaining omega-3s, krill oil is proving to be an even better alternative. May you find that it helps you achieve and maintain optimum health.

Conclusion

Achieving good health does not begin nor does it end with your annual visit to the doctor. While regular checkups are important, they are not the only steps you should take to achieve and maintain physical and mental fitness. As I have stated a number of times throughout this book, it is important to be proactive. I always tell my patients to focus in four areas—diet and nutrition, exercise and flexibility, stress management, and sleep.

Keep your eyes and ears open—try to stay abreast of the latest medical findings and breakthroughs from reputable sources. When faced with a health issue or concern, don't turn your back and hope that it will resolve itself. Seek medical help, ask questions, do your homework. Maintaining such awareness will empower you to make smart, informed decisions regarding your health and the health of your family.

One of the reasons I have written this book is to make you aware of something that I consider to be extremely important in achieving optimal health. Although the vital connection between omega-3 fats and good health has long been supported by the scientific community—and certainly not considered breaking news—the fact that krill oil is a superior source of these nutrients is a relatively recent discovery. It was my goal to raise awareness of this amazing supplement, which, as you have seen, has shown impressive results for maintaining overall good health, as well as for treating a number of common, often debilitating conditions. While I have always been a strong supporter of fish oil as a good source of omega-3s, my extensive research has convinced me that krill oil is an even better choice.

The fact that you have gotten to this portion of this book is very encouraging. But in order to truly benefit from the material you have read, it's time to take the next step. That is, to make krill oil, with its rich abundance of omega-3s, a part of your daily regimen. May it be a small but effective step on your path to better health. I have heard it said that true healthcare reform starts at home, not in Washington. I agree. Good health depends on you. Although it takes a lot of work and discipline, I guarantee your efforts will be well worth it.

Wishing you the best of health,
Dr. Dennis Goodman

References

Introduction

American Heart Association. "Fish and omega-3 fatty acids: AHA recommendation, fish consumption, fish oil, omega-3 fatty acids, and cardiovascular disease."

"Are krill-oil pills as good as fish oil?" ConsumerReports.org. June 2012. http://www.consumerreports.org/cro/2012/05/are-krill-oil-pills-as-good-as-fish-oil/index.htm

Cleland, LG, MJ James, and SM Proudman. "Fish oil: what the prescriber needs to know." *Arthritis Research & Therapy.* 2006; 8(1):202.

"Fish oil." National Institutes of Health. Last modified October 2, 2014. http://www.nlm.nih.gov/medlineplus/druginfo/natural/993.html

Goodman, Dennis. *Magnificent Magnesium: Your Essential Key to a Healthy Heart & More.* Garden City Park, NY: Square One Publishers, 2014.

Halpern, Georges M. *The Inflammation Revolution: A Natural Solution for Arthritis, Asthma, & Other Inflammatory Disorders.* Garden City Park, NY: Square One Publishers, 2005.

Longe, Jacqueline. *The Gale Encyclopedia of Alternative Medicine,* Second Edition. Farmington Hills, MI: Gale Group, 2004.

Masserieh, W. "Health benefits of omega-3 fatty acids from Neptune krill oil." *Lipid Technology.* 2008; 20(5).

Moghadasian, MH. "Advances in dietary enrichment with n-3 fatty acids." *Critical Reviews in Food Science and Nutrition.* 2008; 48(5):402–410.

Natural Standard. "Omega-3 fatty acids, fish oils and alpha-linolenic acid." 2015. http://www.mayoclinic.org/drugs-supplements/omega-3-fatty-acids-fish-oil-alpha-linolenic-acid/background/hrb-20059372

"Omega-3 polyunsaturated fatty acids." http://www.drugs.com/mtm/omega-3-polyunsaturated-fatty-acids.html

Schuchardt, JP, et al. "Incorporation of EPA and DHA into plasma phospholipids in response to different omega-3 fatty acid formulations: a comparative bioavailability study of fish oil vs. krill oil." *Lipids in Health and Disease.* 2011; 10:145.

"Seafood health facts: making smart choices balancing the benefits and risks of seafood consumption." SeafoodHealthFacts.org. http://seafoodhealthfacts.org/

Stoll, Andrew L. *The Omega Connection.* New York: Simon & Schuster, 2001.

"What are fish oils? What are the benefits of fish oils?" MNT Knowledge Center. Last modified September 17, 2014. http://www.medicalnewstoday.com/articles/40253.php

Chapter 1

Bunea, R, K El Farrah, and L Deutsch. "Evaluation of the effects of Neptune krill oil on the clinical course of hyperlipidemia." *Alternative Medicine Review.* 2004; 9(4):420-428.

Callahan, Jack. *The Inflammation Syndrome: Your Nutrition Plan for Great Health, Weight Loss, and Pain-Free Living.* Hoboken, NJ: John Wiley & Sons, 2010.

Cohen, Jay S. *Natural Alternatives to Lipitor, Zocor & Other Statin Drugs.* Garden City Park, NY: Square One Publishers, 2006.

"Fish oil." National Institutes of Health. Last modified October 2, 2014. http://www.nlm.nih.gov/medlineplus/druginfo/natural/993.html

Goodman, Dennis. *Magnificent Magnesium: Your Essential Key to a Healthy Heart & More.* Garden City Park, NY: Square One Publishers, 2014.

Kris-Etherton, PM, et al. "Fish consumption, fish oil, omega-3 fatty acids, and cardiovascular disease." *Circulation.* 2002; 106:2747–2757.

"Mercury: fish consumption advice." Environmental Protection Agency. Last modified December 29, 2014. http://www.epa.gov/mercury/advisories.htm

Mozaffarian, D. "Fish oil and marine omega-3 fatty acids." UpToDate, 2014. www-uptodate-com.ezproxy.med.nyu/contents/fish-oil-and-marine-omega-3-fattyacids

Murray, Michael and Joseph Pizzorno. *The Encyclopedia of Healing Foods.* New York: Atria Books, 2005.

"New insights into how omega-3 fatty acids reduce inflammation also hints at novel disease treatments." University of Pittsburgh Schools of the Health

Sciences. May 3, 2010. http://www.sciencedaily.com/releases/2010/05/100502173503.htm

"Omega-3 fatty acids." University of Maryland Medical Center. Last modified June 24, 2013. http://umm.edu/health/medical/altmed/supplement/omega3-fatty-acids

Schuchardt, JP, et al. "Incorporation of EPA and DHA into plasma phospholipids in response to different omega-3 fatty acid formulations: a comparative bioavailability study of fish oil vs. krill oil." *Lipids in Health and Disease.* 2011; 10:145.

"Seafood & human health." National Oceanic and Atmospheric Administration. www.nmfs.noaa.gov/aquaculture/faqs/faq_seafood_health.html

"Seafood health facts: making smart choices balancing the benefits and risks of seafood consumption." SeafoodHealthFacts.org. http://seafoodhealth facts.org/

Simopoulos, AP. "Omega-3 fatty acids in inflammation and autoimmune diseases." *Journal of the American College of Nutrition.* 2002; 21(6):495–505

Smith, Pamela Wartian. *What You Must Know About Vitamins, Minerals, Herbs & More.* Garden City Park, NY: Square One Publishers, 2008.

Stoll, Andrew L. *The Omega Connection.* New York: Simon & Schuster, 2001.

Ulven, SM, et al. "Metabolic effects of krill oil are essentially similar to those of fish oil but at lower dose of EPA and DHA, in healthy volunteers." *Lipids.* 2011; 46(1):37–46.

Watkins, C. "Krill oil: the next generation source of omega-3s?" *International News on Fats, Oils and Related Materials: INFORM.* September 1, 2007.

"What are fish oils? What are the benefits of fish oils?" MNT Knowledge Center. Last modified September 17, 2014. http://www.medicalnewstoday.com/articles/40253.php

"What is inflammation? What causes inflammation?" MNT Knowledge Center. Last modified September 2, 2014. http://www.medicalnewstoday.com/articles/248423.php

Willerson, JT, and PM Ridker. "Vascular effects of statins: inflammation as a cardiovascular risk factor." *Circulation.* 2004; 109:II2–10.

Chapter 2

Albert, CM, et al. "Blood levels of long-chain n-3 fatty acids and the risk of sudden death." *The New England Journal of Medicine.* 2002; 346:1113–1118.

Cleland, LG, MJ James, and SM Proudman. "Fish oil: what the prescriber needs to know." *Arthritis Research & Therapy.* 2006; 8(1):202.

Corsolini, S, et al. "Occurrence of organochlorine pesticides (OCPs) and their enantiomeric signatures, and concentrations of polybrominated diphenyl ethers (PBDEs) in the Adélie penguin food web, Antarctica." *Environmental Pollution.* 2006; 140:371–382.

Deutsch, L. "Evaluation of the effects of Neptune krill oil on chronic inflammation and arthritic symptoms." *Journal of the American College of Nutrition.* 2007; 26(1):39–48.

"Fish Oil." National Institutes of Health. Last modified October 2, 2014. http://www.nlm.nih.gov/medlineplus/druginfo/natural/993.html

Goodman, Dennis. *Magnificent Magnesium: Your Essential Key to a Healthy Heart & More.* Garden City Park, NY: Square One Publishers, 2014.

"Krill Oil." http://www.drugs.com/krill-oil.html

Kris-Etherton, PM, et al. "Fish consumption, fish oil, omega-3 fatty acids, and cardiovascular disease." *Circulation.* 2002; 106:2747–2757.

Mozaffarian, D. "Fish oil and marine omega-3 fatty acids." UpToDate, 2014. www-uptodate-com.ezproxy.med.nyu/contents/fish-oil-and-marine-omega-3-fattyacids

Mukohpadhyay, R. "The discovery of essential fatty acids: George and Mildred Burr upended the notion that fats only contributed calories in the diet." *The Journal of Biological Chemistry.* November 2012.

Murray, Michael and Joseph Pizzorno. *The Encyclopedia of Healing Foods.* New York: Atria Books, 2005.

"Omega-3 fatty acids." University of Maryland Medical Center. Last modified June 24, 2013. http://umm.edu/health/medical/altmed/supplement/omega3-fatty-acids

"Questions and answers: NIH glucosamine/chondroitin arthritis intervention trial primary study." National Center for Complementary and Integrative Health. Last modified October 2008. https://nccih.nih.gov/research/results/gait/qa.htm

Schuchardt, JP, et al. "Incorporation of EPA and DHA into plasma phospholipids in response to different omega-3 fatty acid formulations: a comparative bioavailability study of fish oil vs. krill oil." *Lipids in Health and Disease.* 2011; 10:145.

Simopoulos, AP. "Omega-3 fatty acids in inflammation and autoimmune diseases." *Journal of the American College of Nutrition.;* 2002: 21(6):495–505

Stubing, D. "Lipid biochemisty of Antarctic euphausiids—energetic adaptations and a critical appraisal of trophic biomarkers." Dissertation zur Erlangung des akademischen Grades eines Doktors der Naturwissenschaften (Dr. rer. nat), Marine Zoologie, Fachbereich Biologie/Chemie, Universitat Bremen, May 2004.

Ulven, SM, et al. "Metabolic effects of krill oil are essentially similar to those of fish oil but at lower dose of EPA and DHA, in healthy volunteers." *Lipids.* 2011; 46(1):37–46.

Watkins, Catherine. "Krill oil: the next generation source of omega-3s?" *International News on Fats, Oils and Related Materials: INFORM.* September 1, 2007.

Williams, C M, and G Burdge. "Long-chain n-3 PUFA: plant v. marine sources." *Proceedings of the Nutrition Society.* 2006; 65:42–50.

Chapter 3

Burri, Lena. *Krill Oil: The Superior Source of Omega-3 Fatty Acids.* Bochum, Germany: Ponte Press, 2013.

"Fish Consumption Advisories." United States Environmental Protection Agency.   http://water.epa.gov/scitech/swguidance/fishshellfish/fish advisories/

Griinari, M, and I Bruheim. "Review of the health benefits of Antarctic krill." Bioriginal Food & Science Corporation, 2015.

Kawaguchi, S, and S Nicol. "Learning about Antarctic krill from the fishery." *Antarctic Science.* 2007; 19(2):219–230.

Schuchardt, JP, et al. "Incorporation of EPA and DHA into plasma phospholipids in response to different omega-3 fatty acid formulations: a comparative bioavailability study of fish oil vs. krill oil." *Lipids in Health and Disease.* 2011; 10:145.

Tou, JC, J Jaczynski, and YC Chen. "Krill for human consumption: nutritional value and potential health benefits." *Nutrition Reviews.* 2007; 65(2):63–77.

Ulven, SM, et al. "Metabolic effects of krill oil are essentially similar to those of fish oil but at lower dose of EPA and DHA, in healthy volunteers." *Lipids.* 2011; 46(1):37–46.

Watkins, Catherine. "Krill oil: the next generation source of omega-3s?" *International News on Fats, Oils and Related Materials: INFORM.* September 1, 2007.

Williams, C M, and G Burdge. "Long-chain n-3 PUFA: plant v. marine sources." *Proceedings of the Nutrition Society.* 2006; 65:42–50.

"World Review of Fisheries and Aquaculture." Highlights of Special Studies Rome. 2008.

Chapter 4

Albert, CM, et al. "Blood levels of long-chain n-3 fatty acids and the risk of sudden death." *The New England Journal of Medicine.* 2002; 346:1113–1118.

Berge, K, et al. "Krill oil supplementation lowers serum triglycerides without increasing low-density lipoprotein cholesterol in adults with borderline high or high triglyceride levels." *Nutrition Research.* 2014; 34(2):126–133.

Bunea, R, K El Farrah, and L Deutsch. "Evaluation of the effects of Neptune krill oil on the clinical course of hyperlipidemia." *Alternative Medicine Review.* 2004; 9(4):420–428.

Burr, ML. "Reflections on the Diet and Reinfarction Trial (DART)." *European Heart Journal Supplements.* 2001; 3(Supplement D):D75–78.

Christensen, JH, et al. "Heart rate variability and fatty acid content of blood cell membranes: a dose-response study with n-3 fatty acids1,2,3." *American Journal of Clinical Nutrition.* 1999; 70(3):331–337.

Dickinson, A. "Benefits of long chain omega-3 fatty acids (EPA, DHA): help protect against heart disease." In *The Benefits of Nutritional Supplements.* Washington, DC: Council for Responsible Nutrition. 2002.

Fosshaug, LE, et al. "Krill oil attenuates left ventricular dilatation after myocardial infarction in rats." *Lipids in Health and Disease.* 2011; 10:245–253.

GISSI-Prevenzione Investigators. "Dietary supplementation with n-3 polyunsaturated fatty acids and vitamin E after myocardial infarction: results of the GISSI-Prevenzione trial." *Lancet.* 1999; 354(9177):447–455.

Goodman, Dennis. *Magnificent Magnesium: Your Essential Key to a Healthy Heart & More.* Garden City Park, NY: Square One Publishers, 2014.

Halpern, Georges M. *The Inflammation Revolution: A Natural Solution for Arthritis, Asthma, & Other Inflammatory Disorders.* Garden City Park, NY: Square One Publishers, 2005.

Hu, FB, et al. "Fish and omega-3 fatty acid intake and risk of coronary heart disease in women." *JAMA.* 2002; 287(14):1815–1821.

Kris-Etherton, PM, et al. "Fish consumption, fish oil, omega-3 fatty acids, and cardiovascular disease." *Circulation.* 2002; 106:2747–2757.

Li, K, et al. "Effect of marine-derived n-3 polyunsaturated fatty acids on c-reactive protein, interleukin 6, and tumor necrosis factor alpha: a meta-analysis." *PloS One.* 2014; 9(2):e88103.

Libby, P. "Atherosclerosis: the new view." *Scientific American.* 2002; 286(5):47–58.

Libby, P, et al. "Inflammation and atherosclerosis." *Circulation.* 2002; 105(9):1135–1143.

Maier, JAM. "Endothelial cells and magnesium: implications in atherosclerosis." *Clinical Science.* 2012; 122(9):397–407.

Maki, KC, et al. "Krill oil supplementation increases plasma concentrations of eicosapentaenoic and docosahexaenoic acids in overweight and obese men and women." *Nutrition Research.* 2009; 29(9):609–615.

Mann, George V, ed. *Coronary Heart Disease: The Dietary Sense and Nonsense.* New York: Veritas Society, 1993.

Micallef, MA, and ML Garg. "Anti-inflammatory and cardioprotective effects of n-3 polyunsaturated fatty acids and plant sterols in hyperlipidemic individuals." *Atherosclerosis.* 2009; 204(2):476–482.

Miles, EA, and PC Calder. "Influence of marine n-3 polyunsaturated fatty acids on immune function and a systematic review of their effects on clinical outcomes in rheumatoid arthritis." *British Journal of Nutrition.* 2012; 107(Suppl 2):S171-S184.

Mozaffarian, D. "Fish oil and marine omega-3 fatty acids." UpToDate, 2014. www-uptodate-com.ezproxy.med.nyu/contents/fish-oil-and-marine-omega-3-fattyacids

Ramprasath, VR, et al. "Enhanced increase of omega-3 index in healthy individuals with response to 4-week n-3 fatty acid supplementation from krill oil versus fish oil." *Lipids in Health and Disease.* 2013, 12:178.

Tandy, S, et al. "Dietary krill oil supplementation reduces hepatic steatosis, glycemia, and hypercholesterolemia in high-fat-fed mice." *Journal of Agricultural and Food Chemistry.* 2009; 57(19):9339–9345.

Ulven, SM, et al. "Metabolic effects of krill oil are essentially similar to those of fish oil but at lower dose of EPA and DHA, in healthy volunteers." *Lipids.* 2011; 46(1):37–46.

Weitz, D, et al. "Fish oil for the treatment of cardiovascular disease." *Cardiology in Review.* 2010; 18(5):258–263.

"What is inflammation? What causes inflammation?" MNT Knowledge Center. Last modified September 2, 2014. http://www.medicalnewstoday.com/articles/248423.php

Willerson, JT, and PM Ridker. "Vascular effects of statins: inflammation as a cardiovascular risk factor." *Circulation.* 2004; 109:II2-10.

Yokoyama, M, et al. "Effects of eicosapentaenoic acid on major coronary events in hypercholesterolaemic patients (JELIS)." *Lancet.* 2007; 369(9567): 1090–1098.

Chapter 5

Barbour, KE, et al. "Prevalence of doctor-diagnosed arthritis and arthritis-attributable activity limitation—United States, 2010–2012." *Morbidity and Mortality Weekly Report (MMWR)*. 2013; 62(44):869–873.

"Cyclosporine (Neoral, Sandimmune, Gengraf)." American College of Rheumatology. Last modified April 2012. https://www.rheumatology.org/Practice/Clinical/Patients/Medications/Cyclosporine_(Neoral,_Sandimmune,_Gengraf)/

Deutsch, L. "Evaluation of the effects of Neptune krill oil on chronic inflammation and arthritic symptoms." *Journal of the American College of Nutrition*. 2007; 26(1):39–48.

Edwards, CJ, and C Cooper. "Early environmental factors and rheumatoid arthritis." *Clinical & Experimental Immunology*. 2006; 143(1):1–5.

Goodman, Dennis. *Magnificent Magnesium: Your Essential Key to a Healthy Heart & More*. Garden City Park, NY: Square One Publishers, 2014.

Halpern, Georges M. *The Inflammation Revolution: A Natural Solution for Arthritis, Asthma, & Other Inflammatory Disorders*. Garden City Park, NY: Square One Publishers, 2005.

Hootman, JM, and CG Helmick. "Projections of US prevalence of arthritis and associated activity limitations." *Arthritis & Rheumatology*. 2006; 54(1):266–229.

Masserieh, W. "Health benefits of omega-3 fatty acids from Neptune krill oil." *Lipid Technology*. 2008; 20(5).

"New insights into how omega-3 fatty acids reduce inflammation also hints at novel disease treatments." University of Pittsburgh Schools of the Health Sciences. May 3, 2010.

http://www.sciencedaily.com/releases/2010/05/100502173503.htm

"Questions and answers: NIH glucosamine/chondroitin arthritis intervention trial primary study." National Center for Complementary and Integrative Health. Last modified October 2008. https://nccih.nih.gov/research/results/gait/qa.htm

Simopoulos, AP. "Omega-3 fatty acids in inflammation and autoimmune diseases." *Journal of the American College of Nutrition*. 2002; 21(6):495–505

"Understanding autoinflammatory diseases." National Institute of Arthritis and Musculoskeletal and Skin Diseases (NIAMS). March 2010. http://www.niams.nih.gov/Health_Info/Autoinflammatory/

"What is inflammation? What causes inflammation?" MNT Knowledge Center. Last modified September 2, 2014. http://www.medicalnewstoday.com/articles/248423.php

Willerson, JT, and PM Ridker. "Vascular effects of statins: inflammation as a cardiovascular risk factor." *Circulation.* 2004; 109:II2-10.

Chapter 6

Burri, Lena. *Krill Oil: The Superior Source of Omega-3 Fatty Acids.* Bochum, Germany: Ponte Press, 2013.

Hawkins, Amy Lee. *What You Must Know About Bioidentical Hormone Replacement Therapy.* Garden City Park, NY: Square One Publishers, 2013.

"LC-PUFA—a guide to health benefits and market trends." *Health and Nutrition.* No. 1. June 2008, Switzerland.

Pick, M. "Balancing your omega-3 fatty acids—essential for health and long life." Women to Women.

http://www.womentowomen.com/inflammation/balancing-your-omega-3-fatty-acids-essential-for-health-and-long-life/

"Premenstrual syndrome (PMS) fact sheet." Office on Women's Health, U.S. Department of Health and Human Services. Last modified December 23, 2014. http://www.womenshealth.gov/publications/our-publications/fact-sheet/premenstrual-syndrome.html

Sampalis, F, et al. "Evaluation of the effects of Neptune krill oil on the management of premenstrual syndrome." *Alternative Medicine Review.* 2003; 8(2):171–179.

Su, KP, et al. "Omega-3 fatty acids for major depressive disorder during pregnancy: results from a randomized, double-blind, placebo-controlled trial." *Journal of Clinical Psychiatry.* 2008; 69 (4):644–651.

Tou, JC, J Jaczynski, and YC Chen. "Krill for human consumption: nutritional value and potential health benefits." *Nutrition Reviews.* 2007; 65(2):63–77.

Chapter 7

Burri, Lena. *Krill Oil: The Superior Source of Omega-3 Fatty Acids.* Bochum, Germany: Ponte Press, 2013.

Carlezon, WA, et al. "Antidepressant-like effects of uridine and omega-3 fatty acids are potentiated by combined treatment in rats."*Biological Psychiatry.* 2005; 57:343–350.

DeMar, JC, et al. "One generation of n-3 polyunsaturated fatty acid deprivation increases depression and aggression test scores in rats." *Journal of Lipid Research.* 2006; 47(1):172–180

"LC-PUFA—a guide to health benefits and market trends." *Health and Nutrition*. No. 1. June 2008, Switzerland.

Lin, PY, SY Huang, KP Su. "A meta-analytic review of polyunsaturated fatty acid compositions in patients with depression." *Biological Psychiatry*. 2010; 68(2):140–147.

Masserieh, W. "Health benefits of omega-3 fatty acids from Neptune krill oil." *Lipid Technology*. 2008; 20(5).

Moghadasian, MH. "Advances in dietary enrichment with n-3 fatty acids." *Critical Reviews in Food Science and Nutrition*. 2008; 48(5):402–410.

Schuchardt, JP, et al. "Incorporation of EPA and DHA into plasma phospholipids in response to different omega-3 fatty acid formulations: a comparative bioavailability study of fish oil vs. krill oil." *Lipids in Health and Disease*. 2011; 10:145.

Su, KP, et al. "Omega-3 fatty acids for major depressive disorder during pregnancy: results from a randomized, double-blind, placebo-controlled trial." *Journal of Clinical Psychiatry*. 2008; 69(4):644–651.

Tou, JC, J Jaczynski, and YC Chen. "Krill for human consumption: nutritional value and potential health benefits." *Nutrition Reviews*. 2007; 65(2):63–77.

Videbech, P, and B Ravnkilde. "Hippocampal volume and depression: a meta-analysis of MRI studies." *The American Journal of Psychiatry*. 2004; 161(11): 1957–1966.

Chapter 8

Balbas, MG, SM Regana, and UP Millet. "Study on the use of omega-3 fatty acids as a therapeutic supplement in treatment of psoriasis." *Journal of Clinical, Cosmetic, and Investigative Dermatology*. 2011; 4:73–77.

Burri, Lena. *Krill Oil: The Superior Source of Omega-3 Fatty Acids*. Bochum, Germany: Ponte Press, 2013.

"Caring for Cancer: Krill Oil." *Alternative Medicine*. Last modified February 2011. https://www.caring4cancer.com/myhealthcenter/tools/knowledgebase/Article.aspx?Hwid=hn-10002454

Fernandez, E. "Lifestyle changes may lengthen telomeres, a measure of cell aging." University of California San Francisco. September 16, 2013.

Goodman, Dennis. *Magnificent Magnesium: Your Essential Key to a Healthy Heart & More*. Garden City Park, NY: Square One Publishers, 2014.

Grimstad, T, et al. "Dietary supplementation of krill oil attenuates inflammation and oxidative stress in experimental ulcerative colitis in rats." *Scandinavian Journal of Gastroenterology*. 2012; 47(1):49–58.

Halpern, Georges M. *The Inflammation Revolution: A Natural Solution for Arthritis, Asthma, & Other Inflammatory Disorders.* Garden City Park, NY: Square One Publishers, 2005.

"LC-PUFA—a guide to health benefits and market trends." *Health and Nutrition.* No. 1. June 2008, Switzerland.

Longe, Jacqueline. *The Gale Encyclopedia of Alternative Medicine,* Second Edition. Farmington Hills, MI: Gale Group, 2004.

Masserieh, W. "Health benefits of omega-3 fatty acids from Neptune krill oil." *Lipid Technology.* 2008; 20(5).

Miles, EA, and PC Calder. "Influence of marine n-3 polyunsaturated fatty acids on immune function and a systematic review of their effects on clinical outcomes in rheumatoid arthritis." *British Journal of Nutrition.* 2012; 107(Suppl 2):S171-S184.

Mozaffarian, D. "Fish oil and marine omega-3 fatty acids." UpToDate, 2014. www-uptodate-com.ezproxy.med.nyu/contents/fish-oil-and-marine-omega-3-fattyacids

"New insights into how omega-3 fatty acids reduce inflammation also hints at novel disease treatments." University of Pittsburgh Schools of the Health Sciences. May 3, 2010. http://www.sciencedaily.com/releases/2010/05/100502173503.htm

SanGiovanni, JP, and EY Chew. "The role of omega-3 long-chain polyunsaturated fatty acids in health and disease of the retina." *Progress in Retinal and Eye Research.* 2005; 24(1):87–138.

Tanalgo, PV, CR Dass, and XQ Su. "Krill oil inhibits proliferation of human colorectal cancer cells." Presented at the 2014 ISSFAL Biennial Congress.

Tou, JC, J Jaczynski, and YC Chen. "Krill for human consumption: nutritional value and potential health benefits." *Nutrition Reviews.* 2007; 65(2):63–77.

"Understanding autoinflammatory diseases." National Institute of Arthritis and Musculoskeletal and Skin Diseases (NIAMS). March 2010. http://www.niams.nih.gov/Health_Info/Autoinflammatory/

"What Is Alzheimer's?" Alzheimer's Association. www.alz.org/alzheimers_disease_what_is_alzheimers.asp

Chapter 9

Beaudoin, A, and G Martin, inventors. "Method of extracting lipids from marine and aquatic animal tissues." United States Patent Number US6800299 B1. October 5, 2004.

Cleland, LG, MJ James, and SM Proudman. "Fish oil: what the prescriber needs to know." *Arthritis Research & Therapy.* 2006; 8(1):202.

"Fish Oil." National Institutes of Health. Last modified October 2, 2014. http://www.nlm.nih.gov/medlineplus/druginfo/natural/993.html

Goodman, Dennis. *Magnificent Magnesium: Your Essential Key to a Healthy Heart & More.* Garden City Park, NY: Square One Publishers, 2014.

Kris-Etherton, PM, et al. "Fish consumption, fish oil, omega-3 fatty acids, and cardiovascular disease." *Circulation.* 2002; 106:2747–2757.

Mozaffarian, D. "Fish oil and marine omega-3 fatty acids." UpToDate, 2014. www-uptodate-com.ezproxy.med.nyu.edu/contents/fish-oil-and-marine-omega-3-fattyacids

"New insights into how omega-3 fatty acids reduce inflammation also hints at novel disease treatments." University of Pittsburgh Schools of the Health Sciences. May 3, 2010. http://www.sciencedaily.com/releases/2010/05/100502173503.htm

O'Connor, Anahad. "What's in your fish oil supplements?" *The New York Times.* January 22, 2014.

"Omega-3 fatty acids." University of Maryland Medical Center. Last modified June 24, 2013. http://umm.edu/health/medical/altmed/supplement/omega3-fatty-acids

Schuchardt, JP, et al. "Incorporation of EPA and DHA into plasma phospholipids in response to different omega-3 fatty acid formulations: a comparative bioavailability study of fish oil vs. krill oil." *Lipids in Health and Disease.* 2011; 10:145.

Smith, Pamela Wartian. *What You Must Know About Vitamins, Minerals, Herbs & More.* Garden City Park, NY: Square One Publishers, 2008.

Tou, JC, J Jaczynski, and YC Chen. "Krill for human consumption: nutritional value and potential health benefits." *Nutrition Reviews.* 2007; 65(2):63–77.

About the Author

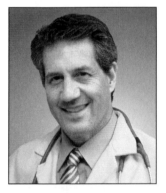

Dr. Dennis Goodman, MD, FACC, gradu-
ated cum laude and with distinction
from the University of Cape Town
Medical School in Cape Town, South
Africa, in 1979. He served his intern-
ship at Grootte Schuur Hospital in
Cape Town, South Africa, and complet-
ed his internal medicine residency at
Montefiore Hospital in Pittsburgh,
Pennsylvania, where he was also Chief
Medical Resident. Dr. Goodman served his cardiology fellowship
at Baylor College of Medicine in Houston, Texas.

Dr. Goodman is board certified in internal medicine, cardiol-
ogy, interventional cardiology, clinical lipidology, critical care,
integrative holistic and integrative medicine, and cardiac CT
imaging. In 1988, he joined Scripps Memorial Hospital in La Jolla,
California, where he served as Chief of Cardiology and Medical
Director of Cardiac Rehabilitation. In 2009 he joined the New York
University cardiology faculty and was appointed Director of
Chest Pain at Bellevue Hospital in New York.

Currently, Dr. Goodman is a Clinical Associate Professor of
Medicine at New York University. He is also a faculty member of
Leon H. Charney Division of Cardiology and Preventative Medi-

cine at NYU, as well as the Director of Integrative Medicine. His area of special interest lies in the prevention, early detection, and treatment of cardiovascular disease with an integrative approach to optimal patient health care.

The author of three books on heart health, Dr. Goodman is a noted international speaker and has been a visiting teaching professor throughout Europe, Asia, South Africa, Israel, and the United Kingdom. His articles have been widely published, and he has appeared on numerous radio and television programs on such major networks as FOX, ABC, CBS, and NBC. Dr. Goodman has been consistently listed among New York's Top Physicians and Cardiologists.

Index

AA. *See* Arachidonic acid.

Acetaminophen, 78–79

Acetylcholine, 42

Acute myocardial infarction. *See* Heart attack.

Addison's disease, as inflammatory condition, 17

ADHD. *See* Attention deficit hyperactivity disorder.

Aging, 114

ALA. *See* Alpha-linolenic acid.

Allergies, as inflammatory conditions, 17

Alpha-linolenic acid (ALA), 10–11, 27

   health benefits of, 10

   sources of, 10-11, 28–29

Alternative Medicine Review, 89

Alzheimer's disease, 114–116

American Academy of Orthopaedic Surgeons, 73

American Cancer Society, 118

American College of Obstetricians and Gynecologists, 85

American Heart Association, 50, 60

American Journal of Clinical Nutrition, The, 95

Angina pectoris, 51–52

Annals of the Rheumatic Diseases, 81

Antidepressants, 88–89, 101–102, 105

Arachidonic acid (AA), 11, 31

Arthritis,

   and benefits of krill oil, 82–83

   and benefits of omega-3s, 81–82

   and inflammation, 82–83

   overview, 69–71

   statistics for, 69

   treating, 77–83

   types of, 71–80

See also Osteoarthritis; Rheumatoid arthritis.

Astaxanthin, 32, 83, 112, 123
  as natural preservative, 38, 44, 83, 109, 130
  health benefits of, 43–44

Asthma, 117–118

Atherosclerosis, 18, 52–53, 60, 61–62

Atherosclerosis, 66

Attention deficit hyperactivity disorder (ADHD), 112–113

Autoimmune disorders, 17–18

Bang, Hans Olaf, 26

Bayley Psychomotor Development Index, 93

Bioavailability, 27, 28, 42

Biologics, 80

Bipolar disorder, 20

Black box warning, 89

Blood-brain barrier, 112

Burr, George, 25

Burr, Mildred, 25

Cancer, 118–119

Carcinogenesis, 119

Cardiac arrest, 53–54

Cardiff University, 82

Cardiopulmonary arrest. *See* Cardiac arrest.

Cardiovascular disease
  and benefits of krill oil, 66–68
  and benefits of omega-3s, 49, 63–66
  as inflammatory condition, 18, 60–62
  overview, 49
  risk factors, 59–60
  statistics for, 49, 50
  studies on, 64–68
  treating, 62–63
  types of, common, 51–59

Cardiovascular health, and connection with omega-3s, 26

CCAMLR. *See* Commission for the Conservation of Antarctic Marine Living Resources.

CDC. *See* Centers for Disease Control.

Celecoxib, 78

Centers for Disease Control (CDC), 69, 72

Cholesterol, 8, 12

Choline, 42–43, 109

Chondroitin sulfate, 80

Circulatory arrest. *See* Cardiac arrest.

Climate change, challenges of, 47

Clinical depression. *See* Depression.

Cod liver oil, 24

Codeine, 79

Cognitive therapy, 100–101

Commission for the Conservation of Antarctic Marine Living Resources (CCAMLR), 46, 47

Congestive heart failure, 18, 54–55

Coronary artery disease. *See* Coronary heart disease.

Coronary heart disease, 55–56

Corticosteroids, 79

Corticotropin-releasing hormone (CRH), 108

COX-1 enzyme. *See* Cyclooxygenase 1.

COX-2 enzyme. *See* Cyclooxygenase 2.

COX-2 inhibitors, 78

C-reactive protein (CRP), 66, 82, 83

CRH. *See* Corticotropin-releasing hormone.

Crohn's disease, 17, 120

Crop and Food Research Institute, 129

CRP. *See* C-reactive protein.

Cyclooxygenase 1 (COX-1), 77, 78

Cyclooxygenase 2 (COX-2), 18–19, 77, 78, 82

Cyclosporine, 80

Cytokines, 76

DART. *See* Diet and Reinfarction Trial

DCRP. *See* Depression Clinical and Research Program.

Dementia, 113–116

Depression, 87
about, 97–99
and benefits of krill oil, 108–109

and benefits of omega-3s, 107–108
causes/risk factors, 99–100
symptoms, 97
treating, 100–102, 105–106

Depression Clinical and Research Program (DCRP), 90, 108

DES. *See* Dry eye syndrome.

Detritus, 40

Developmental ascent, 40

DHA. *See* Docosahexaenoic acid.

Diagnostic and Statistical Manual of Mental Disorders (DSM), 98

Diet and Reinfarction Trial (DART), 64–65

Disease-modifying antirheumatic drugs (DMARDs), 79–80

DMARDs. *See* Disease-modifying antirheumatic drugs.

Docosahexaenoic acid (DHA), 9, 27
and ADHD, 112
and aging, 115
and bioavailoability in fish oil, 42
and bioavailoability in krill oil, 42
and depression, 108–109
and eye health, 122–123
and fetal development, 92
and infant development, 93–94
and joint pain, 81–82

and role in hormone production, 21
health benefits of, 10, 21, 64
in fish oil, 37
in krill oil, 38
sources of, 10, 27
Donald W. Reynolds Cardiovascular Research Center, 60
Dopamine, 86, 87, 103, 104
Dry eye syndrome (DES), 122–123
DSM. *See Diagnostic and Statistical Manual of Mental Disorders.*
Dyerberg, Jørn, 26
Dysmenorrhea, 91

EFAs. *See* Essential fatty acids.
Eicosanoids, 83
Eicosapentaenoic acid (EPA), 9, 27
and aging, 115
and bioavailoability in fish oil, 42
and bioavailoability in krill oil, 42
and cancer, 119
and depression, 108, 109
and eye health, 122–123
and irritable bowel syndrome, 120
and role in hormone production, 21
health benefits of, 10, 21, 64, 81–82
in fish oil, 37

in krill oil, 38
sources of, 10, 27
Endocrine system
about, 19–20
disorders, 20–21
Environmental Protection Agency (EPA), 134
EPA. *See* Eicosapentaenoic acid.
EPA. *See* US Environmental Protection Agency.
Epinephrine, 103–104
Ethyl esters, 36, 37
Euphausia superba krill species, 40

Faroe Islands studies, 93
Fats, dietary
about, 7
monounsaturated, 9
polyunsaturated fats, 9
saturated, 8
trans, 8
unsaturated, 8–9
See also Omega-3 fatty acids; Omega-6 fatty acids.
FDA. *See* US Food and Drug Administration.
Fetal development, 92, 112
Fish
and contaminant considerations, 33–34
as source of omega-3s, 32
farmed, 33, 35
Fish oil
and cancer, 119
and cardiovascular disease, 64–67

and contaminant
considerations, 128–129

and digestibility issues, 37

and form of omega-3s, 37

and inflammatory bowel
disease, 120

and lupus, 117

and premenstrual syndrome,
90

and psoriasis, 121

bioavailability of, 37, 42

compared to krill oil, 38, 41,
42, 44, 67, 89, 119, 130, 139

first pharmaceutical, 24

FOS. *See* Friends of the Sea.

Free radicals, 43

Friends of the Sea (FOS), 46

Fuster, Valentin, 60

GABA. *See* Gamma-
aminobutyric acid.

Gamma-aminobutyric acid
(GABA), 104

Gamma-linolenic acid (GLA), 11

Genetically modified organisms
(GMOs), 30

GISSI-Prevenzione Trial, 64

GLA. *See* Gamma-linolenic acid.

Global Organization for EPA and
DHA Omega-3 (GOED), 134

Glucosamine, 80

GMOs. *See* Genetically
modified organisms.

GOED. *See* Global Organization
for EPA and DHA Omega-3.

Halpern, Georges M., 75–76

Harvard University, 60

HDLs. *See* High-density
lipoproteins, 8

Heart attack, 56–57

Heart disease
and inflammation, 18, 61–62

current view of, 60–62

treating, 62–63

*Heart Disease and Stroke
Statistics—2013 Update*, 50

Hemorrhagic stroke, 58

High blood pressure, 57

High-density lipoproteins
(HDLs), 8, 12

HLAs. *See* Human leukocyte
antigens.

Holman, Ralph, 25

Hormone production
and role of omega-3s, 21

Hormones
and premenstrual syndrome,
86–87

role of, 19–20

See also Depression;
Endocrine system;
Neurotransmitters.

Human leukocyte antigens
(HLAs), 76

Hypertension. *See* High blood
pressure.

Hyperthyroidism, 20

Hypothyroidism, 20

IBD. *See* Inflammatory bowel
disease.

Ibuprofen, 77
Indiana University, 118
Infant development, 93–94
Inflammation, 15–19, 60–62
    acute, 15–16, 61
    and omega-3s, 18–19
    chronic, 16–18, 60, 61,
        116–121, 118–119
    See also Autoimmune
        disorders; Heart disease.
Inflammation Revolution, The
    (Halpern), 75–76
Inflammatory bowel disease
    (IBD), 119–120
Interleukin-1, 76, 82
Interleukin-6, 66
International Journal of Cancer,
    119
International Journal of
    Opthalmology, 122
Ischemia, 51
Ischemic stroke, 58
ISSFAL Biennial Congress, 119

Japan EPA Lipid Intervention
    Study (JELIS), 65
JELIS. *See* Japan EPA Lipid
    Intervention Study
Joint replacement surgery, 81
Joints, about, 70
Journal of Biological Chemistry,
    25
Journal of Clinical, Cosmetic, and
    Investigational Dermatology,
    121

Journal of the American College of
    Nutrition, 82
Journal of the American Medical
    Association, 63, 115

Keyes, Ancel, 26
Krill, 9, 37–38
    about, 39–41
    and placement on food
        chain, 38
    components of, 44
    harvesting and sustainability
        of, 44, 46–47
Krill oil,
    and arthritis, 82–83
    and ADHD, 112–113
    and cardiovascular disease,
        67–68
    and dementia, 116
    and depression, 108–109
    and dysmenorrhea, 91
    and extraction-method
        development, 45
    and form of omega-3s, 38
    and mood, 90
    and premenstrual syndrome,
        90
    and psoriasis, 121
    and safety issues, 134
    benefits of, 48, 67–68
    bioavailability of, 38, 42
    buying guidelines for,
        130–133
    cautions and
        contraindications, 135

compared to fish oil, 38, 41–42, 44, 48, 67, 89, 119, 130, 139

   serving guidelines for, 130–131

   storage guidelines for, 133

LabDoor, 128, 129

LDLs. *See* Low-density lipoproteins, 8

Leflunomide, 80

Libby, Peter, 60

Linoleic acid, 11

Lipid bilayer, 12–13

Lipids in Health and Disease, 67

Low-density lipoproteins (LDLs), 8, 12

Lupus, 17, 117

Lupus Foundation of American, 117

Lymphocytes, 76

Manic depression. *See* Bipolar disorder.

MAOIs. *See* Monoamine oxidase inhibitors.

Marine Stewardship Council (MSC), 46

Massachusetts General Hospital, 90, 108

Mayo Clinic, 72

Menopause, 94–95

Mercury, presence in fish, 33, 34

Microalgae, 32

Möller, Peter, 24

Monoamine oxidase inhibitors (MAOIs), 101, 105

Monounsaturated fats, 9

MSC. *See* Marine Stewardship Council.

n-3 fatty acids. *See* Omega-3 fatty acids.

n-6 fatty acids. *See* Omega-6 fatty acids.

Narcotics, 79

National Center for Health Statistics, 69

National Health Interview Survey, 69

National Institute of Arthritis and Musculoskeletal and Skin Diseases (NIAMS), 75, 76

National Institutes of Health (NIH), 76, 107

Nature of Chemical Biology, 19

Neptune Technologies & Bioressources, 45, 113

Neurotransmitters, 86–87, 103–104, 108

NIAMS. *See* National Institute of Arthritis and Musculoskeletal and Skin Diseases.

NIH. *See* National Institutes of Health.

Nonsteroidal anti-inflammatory drugs (NSAIDs), 77–78, 91

Norepinephrine, 86, 87, 103–104

NSAIDs. *See* Nonsteroidal anti-inflammatory drugs.

Nurses Health Study, 65–66

OA. *See* Osteoarthritis.
Oleic acid, 11
Omega-3 deficiency
  symptoms of, 126
  treating, 126–129
Omega-3 fatty acids, 9, 10–11
  and ADHD, 112–113
  and aging, 114–115
  and arthritis, 81–82
  and asthma, 118
  and cancer, 119
  and cardiovascular disease,
    26, 49, 63–68
  and dementia, 114–116
  and depression, 90, 107–109
  and dysmenorrhea, 90
  and fetal development, 92
  and hormone imbalance, 21
  and lupus, 117
  and postpartum depression,
    94
  and psoriasis, 121–122
  and ratio to omega-6s, 11
  and role in cells, 12–14,
  and role in hormone
    production, 13, 21
  and role in inflammation,
    18–19
  forms of in marine oils,
    36–37
  health benefits of, 6–7, 10,
    13–14, 19, 21, 64
  history of, 24

  See also Alpha-linolenic acid;
    Docosahexaenoic acid;
    Eicosapentaenoic acid;
    Omega-3 fatty acids,
    sources of.
Omega-3 fatty acids, sources of
  animal-based, 31–32
  ocean-based, 32–34
  plant-based, 28–30
Omega-3 status, determining,
  125–127
Omega-6 fatty acids, 9, 10, 27
  and ratio to omega-3s, 11
  health benefits of, 11
  See also Arachidonic acid;
    Gamma-linolenic acid;
    Linoleic acid.
Omega-9 fatty acids, 11–12
  health benefits of, 11
Organic foods, 30
Osteoarthritis (OA)
  about, 71
  causes/risk factors, 72–73
  symptoms, 71
  See also Arthritis.
Oxycodone, 79

PCBs. *See* Polychlorinated
  biphenyls.
Phosphatidyl-choline, 42–43
Phospholipid bilayer, 12–13
Phospholipids, 13, 36, 37, 38,
  41–42, 67
Phytoplankton, 32, 40
Plankton, 32

Plaque, atherosclerotic, 60

Plaque, vulnerable, 56, 60

Plaque buildup
   and atherosclerosis, 52
   and inflammation, 18

Plaque psoriasis, 121

PMDD. *See* Premenstrual
   dysphoric disorder.

PMS. *See* Premenstrual
   syndrome.

Polychlorinated biphenyls
   (PCBs), 33, 36, 134

Polyunsaturated fats, 9

Postpartum depression, 94

Pregnancy, 91
   See also Fetal development;
   Infant development;
   Postpartum depression.

Premenstrual dysphoric
   disorder (PMDD), 86, 88

Premenstrual syndrome (PMS)
   about, 85–87
   and benefits of krill oil,
      89–90
   and benefits of omega-3s,
      89–90
   causes, 86, 87
   symptoms, 85–86
   treatments, 87–89

Preterm birth, 93

*Proceedings of the National
   Academy of Sciences,* 18

Prostaglandins, 18, 77

Psoriasis, 17, 121-122

Psoriatic arthritis, as
   inflammatory condition, 17

Psychodynamic therapy, 101

Psychotherapy, 100–101

Queen Mary, University of
   London, 119

RA. *See* Rheumatoid arthritis.

*Reviews in Obstetrics &
   Gynecology,* 91

Rheumatoid arthritis (RA)
   about, 18, 74–76
   causes/risk factors,76–77
   symptoms, 74, 75
   See also Arthritis.

Rheumatoid nodules, 75

Royal College of Surgeons, 108

Saturated fats, 8

*Scandinavian Journal of
   Gastroenterology,* 120

Selective serotonin reuptake
   inhibitors (SSRIs), 88, 89,
   10–102

Serotonin, 87, 104

Serotonin and norepinephrine
   reuptake inhibitors (SNRIs),
   101, 102

Seven Country Study, 26

SNRIs. *See* Serotonin and
   norepinephrine reuptake
   inhibitors.

SSRIs. *See* Selective serotonin
   reuptake inhibitors.

St. John's wort, 106

Stroke, 58–59

Sudden cardiac arrest. *See* Cardiac arrest.

Sudden cardiac death. *See* Cardiac arrest.

Synovial fluid, 70

Synovium, 70, 76

Talk therapy. *See* Psychotherapy,

TCAs. *See* Tricyclic antidepressants.

Telomeres, 114–115

TNF. *See* Tumor necrosis factor.

Trans fats, 8

Tricyclic antidepressants (TCAs), 101, 102

Triglycerides, 14, 40
in marine oil, 36, 37, 40–41

Trimethylglycine, 42–43

Tumor necrosis factor (TNF), 76, 82

Ulcerative colitis, 120

Université Laval, 95

University of California in San Francisco, 115

University of Pittsburgh Schools of Health Sciences, 19

Unsaturated fats, 8–9

US Environmental Protection Agency (EPA), 33, 36

US Food and Drug Administration (FDA), 89, 92, 134

USP Dietary Supplement Verification Program, 129

Vasculitis, as inflammatory condition, 18

Victoria University, 119

Vulnerable plaque, 56, 60, 61

Wellwise,org, 131

WHO. *See* World Health Organization.

World Health Organizaton (WHO), 134